LEARNING
TO LISTEN

By T. Berry Brazelton, MD, and Others

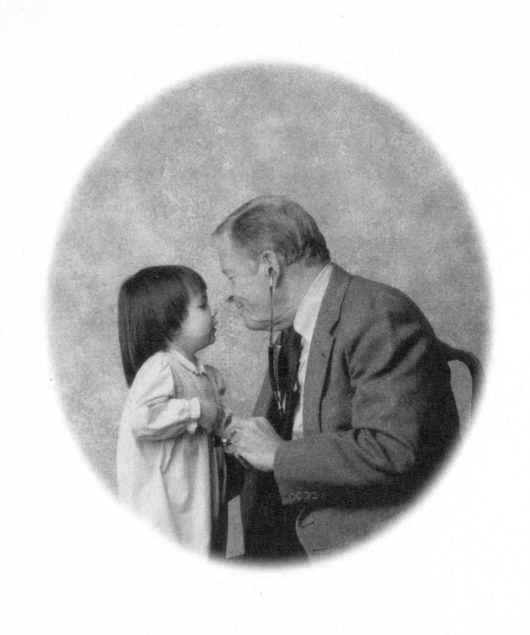

T. Berry Brazelton, MD

LEARNING TO LISTEN

A Life Caring for Children

A Merloyd Lawrence Book
DA CAPO PRESS
A Member of the Perseus Books Group

Frontispiece photo: © Hornick-Rivlin

Designed by Trish Wilkinson
Set in 11.5 point Goudy Old Style by The Perseus Books Group

Library of Congress Cataloging-in-Publication Data

Brazelton, T. Berry, 1918-
    Learning to listen : a life caring for children / T. Berry Brazelton, MD.
        pages cm
    "A Merloyd Lawrence Book."
    Includes index.
    ISBN 978-0-7382-1667-6 (hardcover : alk. paper) — ISBN 978-0-7382-1668-3
(e-book) 1. Brazelton, T. Berry, 1918– 2. Child development. 3. Child
psychologists—United States—Biography. I. Title.
RJ131.B697 2013
618.92'89—dc23

Published as a Merloyd Lawrence Book by Da Capo Press
A Member of the Perseus Books Group
www.dacapopress.com

Da Capo Press books are available at special discounts for bulk purchases in the U.S. by corporations, institutions, and other organizations. For more information, please contact the Special Markets Department at the Perseus Books Group, 2300 Chestnut Street, Suite 200, Philadelphia, PA 19103, or call (800) 810-4145, ext. 5000, or e-mail special.markets@perseusbooks.com.

10 9 8 7 6 5 4 3 2 1

*To my lovely wife, Christina, who accompanied me
through most of this—for sixty-four years now.
And to my four wonderful children,
including Christina II, who helped read and edit
so much of this memoir.*

Contents

Photos following page 118

ONE

Waco to Princeton:
"Berry's So Good with Babies"

Waco, where I was born on May 10, 1918, to Pauline Battle
Brazelton and Thomas Berry Brazelton, is known as the
"Heart of Texas." It was a small town in those days, and
to the residents' dismay, it has stayed a small town. When I was
little, Waco had one tall building. I used to dream about it falling
on our house and killing all of us. No one could entirely convince
me that we were too many blocks away.

There were three distinct social classes in Waco: white, black,
and Mexican American. White people owned and ran everything.
Black people did all of the domestic work, and Mexican Americans
did the rest. The black woman who primarily raised me from age
two on was our cook, my beloved Annie May. She had a son my
age with whom I was never allowed to play. In our Texas town,
there was openly expressed prejudice about how "uppity" blacks
could be. In school black children were treated differently, as if

they were expected to fail. As for the Mexican American children, few even got to school. In my memory, those few wore ragged, dirty clothes, and we white children were taught early on to shun them. I remember wanting to play with them and resenting these societal barriers. Looking back I wonder whether part of my life's work may have been compensation for the deep hurts and prejudices I saw inflicted on many children in this small, ultraconservative town.

My Parents

My father, Thomas Berry Brazelton, was born and raised in Waco. His family owned lumberyards throughout Texas. After attending the Virginia Military Institute for one year, he headed to Princeton. While he was there, he lettered in football, track, crew, and swimming. His real love was diving, and he was an intercollegiate champion at Princeton in 1914.

Dad was a rebel in Waco. Though a member of the conservative city council, he advocated for equal rights for blacks and Mexican Americans. His father, my grandfather Ba, famous as a liberal before him, tried to prevent the lynching of a young black boy who was on trial for allegedly raping a white woman. We were a marked family in a religious, right-wing town. As I remember, when I was in preschool, the Ku Klux Klan burned a cross in front of our house. Dad would disappear because they often came looking for him. Mother would fend them off. Annie May would gather my brother, Chuck, and me and climb under the bed in the back room as if that might shield us.

During prohibition in the late 1920s, Dad also took an independent position. I remember hearing a bang in our cellar as we sat upstairs at dinner. His face paled and he said, "Oh my God! Now don't any of you go into the cellar until we hear twenty-nine more bangs." He was making homemade beer, and it was exploding. Dad was high-strung because of hyperthyroidism and had to have his thyroid removed in 1925 by Dr. George Crile in Cleveland, Ohio. Before that he had been terribly difficult to live with. At one point we went to a resort in Arkansas to try to calm him down. Once my father was on medication, he was quiet and subdued, but Mother remained preoccupied by his illness and was often hard to reach. In an effort to make everyone happier, I stole a toy train from a shop to give to Chuck. Mother made me return it and apologize to the owner. I was devastated.

My mother was a gallant and strong-minded woman. Gifted as a pianist, she was sent away to the conservatory in Cleveland and subsequently performed as a solo pianist with the Fort Worth symphony. At some point in her teens she was diagnosed with TB (as were so many in those days) and sent to a spa in Asheville, North Carolina, for the summer. One night while playing the piano, she was approached by my father, then a sprightly Princetonian. "Can you play any Gershwin?" Back then this was new and daring music. She played for him and their courtship began. Marriage was inevitable. My parents were married in Waco but traveled back to Asheville for their honeymoon. I'm told I was conceived at the Manor Hotel in Asheville. Though my father had wanted to settle in New York, having been offered the equivalent of a seat on the stock exchange, his father wanted him to return to Waco to help run the lumber business. In those days, sons and daughters were expected to accept their family's wishes. I am not sure that he ever fully recovered from his longing to be on the East Coast. My mother sensed his anguish at being brought back to Waco and did her best to support him. She gave up her piano for golf. They played together every day. Family meals were about the shots they should have made but didn't. They were both top seeded, so tournaments were the highlights of their lives. I've hated golf ever since and have never played it.

When I was born during the First World War, my father was away training on the East Coast. I was nine months old when he first saw me. I was told my mother was waiting in a long line at the station, dressed in her best new suit. I was in her arms, probably fingering her nose, her mouth, pulling on her earrings. A long line of uniformed and medaled men came off the train. My father would have come down the platform, half running, in his well-cut uniform with its captain's bars. He was handsome—not his face and his prominent nose but in the athletic way he carried himself. Apparently he rushed up, hugging both of us at once and took me abruptly out of my mother's arms. "Little Berry!" he shouted as he squeezed me in a big hug. As the story goes, I began to cry, louder and louder. What right did this absolute stranger have to take me from my mother's familiar and warm chest? What right did he have to yell at me and squeeze me? I'm told I wailed louder and louder, in the chaos of all these reuniting families. My father was no doubt stunned. "He doesn't like me!" he said to my mother as he handed me back.

The story rings true to me as I've grown to understand both the acute awareness of nine-month-old babies at the peak of stranger anxiety and the hypersensitivity of a new father as he tries to connect with his baby for the first time. Had my father known to wait until I reached out for him, our relationship might have been different from the first. Reflecting on this story later on sparked my interest in establishing a rapport with fathers-to-be during pregnancy and preparing them for times when their relationship with the baby may be strained, so that they can understand the baby's behavior and not feel hurt or resentful. In my practice, I've sought to capture fathers for their babies from the first.

The chance in later years to watch fathers who weren't present for the first several months of their child's life confirmed the importance of a father's early experiences with his baby. It isn't easy for a parent to catch up with the milestones of development; the stresses around a new baby—the diapering, the burping, the unresolved crying, the mistakes—all become positive steps in the family's growth. A father who has to suffer through these initial vicissitudes is setting down layers of attachment to his baby.

My father missed out on this early relationship and, perhaps as a result, always seemed pretty distant, even wary of me. I'm sure he loved me but I never really knew him. My mother fostered that distance with what I now see as unconscious "gatekeeping." In my work I've learned that everyone who cares deeply about a baby is in competition for that baby: parents with each other, grandparents who feel "if only they'd do it my way," caregiver and parent, parent and teacher, coach and parent. It's an inevitable reaction and part of attachment. Since my mother had been sole parent through my early infancy, she believed she knew me better. She probably corrected my father whenever he tried to take any responsibility for me, and, as a result, he may have given up early. I have learned that, by alerting adults who care about the same baby to this gatekeeping tendency, they are less at its mercy. Otherwise, they are bound to try to shut the other adult out. When I was older, I interpreted my father's tentativeness as disappointment. Now I am able to see it more clearly. He always professed pride in me but was distant. Remoteness may have been an incentive to me to make him proud, but it also fueled my ambitions. But we were never really friends. He actually seemed closer to my peers than to me.

Swimming and diving continued to be important to my father. He used to take me and my best friend, Jesse Milam, out to the Fish Pond country club's pool for diving lessons. He spent all of his time encouraging and praising Jesse. Yet when I'd try and even succeed in completing the same maneuvers, he was silent, without comment, as if he had expected me to learn from the teaching he gave my friend. Feeling that I couldn't please him, I became clumsier, and he would ignore me even more. To me, locker rooms smelled of sweat and danger. Perhaps the danger I felt was due to the competitive atmosphere. I dreaded going with him and have never been comfortable in clubs since. He wanted to show me off, but I must have made a poor showing. We slid right past each other in our clumsy efforts to connect as father and son. As an adult I missed out on the chance to get to know him better, for he died after my first year of medical school. Years later, when my youngest daughter asked me about her grandfather, I couldn't answer. I didn't know much about who he was as a person.

Minding the Cousins

At every family event, and there were many, I was put in charge of all nine first cousins while aunts and uncles and grandparents prepared for the big dinner. In order to please my grandmother, whom I called Bama, I became adept at handling many small children at once. I could keep them amused and safe and keep them from crying for up to two hours at a time. A miraculous feat, I realize today! Only ten or eleven years old myself, my relative seniority nevertheless dominated them, and they didn't dare not mind me. I learned something else that has served me well over the years: to study children's behavior in order to understand them as individuals. I could look at a face and tell you when one of my cousins was getting hungry rather than dizzy in the rocking swing. I learned to sing to them, to read to them, and to anticipate their meltdowns. Bama used to say, "Berry's so good with babies." Whenever I hear that today, I hear her voice. I've never been as proud of any other accolade. She pointed the way to my becoming a pediatrician and observer of infant and child behavior.

My Brother

My first memory of my only sibling was his birth two and a half years after mine. Churchill Jones Brazelton, whom we called Chuck, was born, as I was, at our house on Gorman Avenue in Waco. My mother was reluctant to give up anything as important as childbirth to a hospital setting. Hospitals were for illness, not for anything that could be done at home. My tonsils were extracted on our kitchen table when I was five. For an earache, my eardrums were punctured at home, without anesthesia. Why have a baby in the hospital?

During the birth, my father sat with me on the porch awaiting the doctor's arrival. The house was quiet. There were no groans, no crying out with labor pains that I can remember. My father, dressed for work in his suit and tie, fidgeted restlessly beside me. Unused to his company, I sat primly by his side—both of us waiting. It seemed endless.

Finally the doctor drove up in his Model T Ford. He extracted his black bag and marched with dignity and assurance past us into the house. "You boys stay here." From that moment, I've never wanted a black doctor's bag because I associate them with my brother's birth and my resentment of him. (My doctor's bag is brown and to this day sits by the front door.) In a short while, there was a piercing infant wail from the back bedroom. "It's over!" shouted my father as he rushed into the house, leaving me alone on the porch. I cringed but didn't move. Would they come back to get me? After an endless time, the doctor returned with his black bag. He gave me what seemed to be a pitying look and said, "You're lucky, you have a lovely little brother. His name is Churchill. Go on in and see him!" I remembered creeping into the house, peeping into the bedroom where my mother was lying in bed, barely awake. My father was sitting in the only chair, exhausted. The nurse midwife who had been with my mother throughout her labor and had directed the delivery was straightening up the bedroom. My new little brother was wrapped up like a mummy and lying quietly in his special little crib next to the bed. I felt as if I must watch this without making a noise. No one had remembered me. I stood alone in the doorway, quiet, afraid to speak. I'll never forget that empty feeling.

It was not an auspicious beginning for my relationship with Chuck. But it got worse. He was so "cute." He was roly-poly most of our childhood. Eminently squeezable. And I wanted terribly to squeeze him but hard. He had a turned-up nose, wavy blonde hair, and a merry, bewitching smile.

I hated him. And in truth we never got to know one another. My mother kept us apart, keeping Chuck to herself. Again, she was gatekeeping without realizing it. I have no memory of playing with him but many memories of fighting with him. We argued about anything and everything, yelling at each other until Mother would yell louder and tell us to stop. Mother always blamed me for the fighting, even when Chuck started it. Did he do it for the attention and, if so, whose? He already had Mother's. Was this an attempt to have as intense a relationship with me as with our mother? But that did not happen. Even at Princeton, where our enrollments overlapped, we had nothing in common and therefore interacted very little. I don't even know what he did there.

When he was born, Bama told my mother, "Chuck will never live up to Berry." This statement aggravated my mother, who subsequently began a lifelong job of spoiling and overprotecting him. She hovered over him in a way that did not allow him to make his own choices about anything. She hand-fed him until he was four. Toilet training and the other important steps in childhood were further occasions for her excessive attention. It left him too dependent on her, and I believe he paid a terrible price for it later in his life.

Chuck was drafted into the army in 1940 and never finished Princeton. He went to Germany, and I was told that he was the first lieutenant to go into Hitler's office after his suicide. He brought home important relics from Hitler's office, which I still have and plan to donate to the Holocaust Museum. After four years in the army, Chuck moved to Paris, where he became an expert on French antiques. Of course, Mother went to visit him there. She and Chuck were more like friends than mother and son. Her visits to me and my family around that time were neither easy nor affectionate. She was uncomfortable with my new wife and had no idea about what my work entailed. Although I think she was proud of my accomplishments, she never expressed that pride.

After Paris, Chuck went to New Orleans and from there to New York City, where he became a well-known collector and dealer. Looking back, I think my mother's overprotection made independent life hard for him. He became an alcoholic. From then on, he depended on her to rescue him from the crises of an alcoholic's life. Even though she went to Al-Anon and learned about enabling, she could not help but continue to try to save him. As for our relationship, Chuck and I came together when he was fifty. We had several years to relate as brothers, though much of that time I was taking care of him and supporting him financially. My children remember frequent calls from New York saying that Chuck had been found drunk and was in Bellevue or needed to go to rehab. When Mother died in 1976, Chuck was undone. He died in 1980 at age sixty from alcoholism. My mother had suffered greatly over his problems, and it was hard for me to watch. I came to realize that my mother's life-long hovering was a sign of misguided passion. One of the more important goals of my pediatric practice has been to help parents channel their passions in a constructive direction, to face problems early on, not waiting until after a child has already failed. I'm also aware that my use of the word *hovering* is pejorative and damning and that it is a judgment leveled at my mother. At the same time it is a useful concept for anyone trying to understand the effects of overprotection and to devise ways of warning overprotective parents of the dangers for their child's subsequent futures. Watching my mother and Chuck certainly gave me insight for my preventive work: our current generation of two-career parents is likely to hover out of guilt at not being at home enough with their children.

Annie May

My caregiver when I was little was a wonderful, ample black woman named Annie May. She lived in the small servant's house behind our house in Waco. She was in her forties and had no husband—just lots of "visitors" to the house out back. Annie May was always there when I came home from school. She always said, "Hello, little Berry! I'm glad you're here. Now, how about some milk and a donut?" She was also our cook during my childhood. I loved her.

Annie May always made me laugh and feel cared for. We giggled every afternoon. I told her my troubles. She told me some of hers. She loved my younger brother, but she loved me openly. She was our main source of security as well as our disciplinarian. After school Mother was always out, often playing golf with my father. When anyone came to visit Annie May, I was jealous. I didn't want to share her. Once, when I was four, I was dressed up and called in to greet Mother's club of stylish ladies. They oohed and aahed, then asked me cutely, "And who do you love best in all the world?" "Annie May," I chirped. My mother's face fell, and I ran out of the room.

When I was sent to preschool, I felt torn away from Annie May, and, with each step in my ventures away from home, I felt a bit more separated from her. Because I wasn't sure she could read, I never wrote her letters from boarding school or college. But I would rush into the kitchen when I got back. She could read my face and we would just pick up where we left off.

After my father died and our circumstances changed, Annie May went to work for another family in Waco. I kept in touch with her there until she died in 1986. I felt devastated and wished that I could have brought her north with me to live.

Montessori

At four, I was sent to a Montessori school. This had been started by a Mrs. Alice Greenhill, who, farsighted for Waco, went to Italy to train under Maria Montessori. Montessori had been a physician in Rome but soon became involved in children's learning. She gave up her medical practice to become a teacher of teachers. One of her important insights was that children learned from "within" much more than they learned from "without." In order to reach each child, she developed a way of observing so as to respond to the individuality of each one. She trained teachers to watch and listen and to trust their observations of each child's temperament, learning style, and desire to learn. For example, she'd urge a teacher to watch a child with a puzzle and not to help her unless she became overwhelmed. She described how, after a child had struggled to solve the puzzle, one could watch her face as she finally mastered it. The glorious recognition of "I did it myself!" showed learning from within. This recognition by Dr. Montessori was twenty to thirty years ahead of Jean Piaget, who later called it the child's "inner feedback cycle" and labeled it the most powerful force of learning. I use their theories to help parents see both their child's struggles and ultimate successes in each stage of development and to urge them to hold off long enough to let the child "do it myself." That sense is a powerful driver of the development of the central nervous system.

I was lucky to be admitted to Mrs. Greenhill's school. It was right across the street. Four of us went to preschool together and became fast friends. After this early exposure to the excitement of "inner learning," we left Montessori after two years and entered first grade at the age of six. We were kept together all the way through school, jumping grades twice, and ended up graduating at the ages of fifteen and sixteen. All four of us were intellectually way ahead of our physical development, and this disconnect cost us emotionally. As the smallest and least developed of all my classmates, it was a terrible burden to my self-esteem to be the last one chosen for every team. No one wanted me on their side. They had begun to grow and develop, to have smelly feet and underarm hair, at least two years before I did. Even if I'd been an athletic star, I'd have had trouble with other boys my age. But I wasn't athletic.

I was smart. I ended up as salutatorian, which didn't contribute to my popularity.

As an adult, I realize what a fine foundation Mrs. Greenhill laid in kindergarten. In contrast, reflecting upon my later school years convinced me that precocity in any area could have a cost in other areas of development. In areas other than schoolwork, I was always seeking reassurance that I could fit in. Although individual differences in children's abilities should be respected as early as possible, precocity in some areas must not overshadow the areas that are underdeveloped.

Nearly Saved

My mother was a fervent Presbyterian whose credo was to think of others before thinking of oneself. She saw to it that on Sunday we attended seven hours of church. I haven't been in church since childhood as a result. My father, however, did not join her in her beliefs and never once came to services with us. Mother believed strongly in all the religious doctrine, especially the part that predicted doom around every corner and required preparedness for disaster at the same time one was enjoying good fortune. In her mind and in what she taught me, the only way to forestall doom's arrival was to work hard for less privileged people. I took this to heart and at the age of eight wanted to be a missionary in Africa in order to give people there better lives.

When I was six, a traveling evangelist named Gypsy Smith came to town. His visit was anticipated eagerly in our otherwise dull world. My mother took Chuck and me to his evening service. Gypsy Smith was flamboyant and exciting as he wooed the audience with his face, his voice, and his flying hands. He was much more convincing than any preacher I'd heard before, especially at the First Presbyterian Church. I was mesmerized. As he invoked the Lord's blessing, he waved his arms, he strutted, and he spoke in a loud, passionate voice. He urged us all to repent our sins and to come forward for redemption during the next hymn. "Just walk up the aisle with your hand out and your souls open. Gypsy Smith and the Lord together will redeem you. Your sins will vanish." I thought about my major sin, cringing at the thought of my deep hatred for my little brother. Could Gypsy Smith be my salvation?

As the organ started up, Gypsy Smith marched back and forth in front of the congregation, calling out to us to "come up and be saved" from our sins. I slid out of my pew and made my way up the aisle to where Gypsy was and gave myself up to be saved. He didn't look at me but past me to the adults who came up behind me. Thinking he couldn't see me because I was small, I pulled on his robe. He looked down and with a look of disdain said, "Get away from me, kid." It şent me crying back to my seat. There would be no redemption that day. And, because of Gypsy Smith, I gave up my dream of being a missionary.

Animal Doctor

Adolescence seemed pretty frightening to me. I turned inward and to my animals for an understanding of the changes I was going through. I had ducks, chickens, rabbits, and my dearest friend, a German shepherd, Smokey. Smokey followed me everywhere. He watched me, listened to me, and followed my directions without my having to train him. He was the favorite of all the newsboys in Waco because he'd rush up to pick up a paper if they missed the porch. He'd carry it up on the porch, deposit it, then return to the newsboy, wagging his tail furiously and looking for his approval. I don't know how I could have faced my own delayed adolescence without him and the rest of my menagerie. I read Dr. Dolittle books and tried to talk to my animals as he did. I learned that their behavior was their language, an insight that has served me all of my professional life. I thought I could talk to them and they to me. When one of my chickens fell off her perch and broke her leg, I mended it by attaching a splint made out of a Popsicle stick. I talked to her all the way through my procedure. I believed that she looked up at me with gratitude after I'd splinted her leg. That confirmed my decision to become a doctor. The leg mended. The chicken would even follow me around the yard afterward. It was a wonderful, heady feeling. I was no longer at the mercy of my peers' image of me as a wimp. My animals trusted me.

When the rabbits produced babies, it became obvious that we'd have to sell or eat some of them. Of course, I couldn't bear to do either. Thank heaven I had a friend next door, an older lady, Mrs. Wood. She offered to take the surplus rabbits off my hands, so I'd have no awful decision to make. In retrospect, I'm sure she ate them, but I didn't have to watch or participate. Mrs. Wood became another surrogate mother to me as we talked about our animals and shared the best way of raising them. She treated me as an equal.

My animals thrived. The ducks and chickens produced eggs. I learned to tell when the rabbits were pregnant by the way they began to walk—to clump rather than dance with their hind legs. Ducks and chickens seemed to act more arrogant just before they laid an egg. The laying was painful, but they seemed to go through it stoically in order to crow about it afterward—a wonderful transition to watch. Smokey and my animals were a great introduction to the facts of life. My father never talked to me about the birds and the bees. No one did. The only talk about sex we had was when he offered the warning typical of that time, not to mastur-bate, "because it would make you go crazy."

Texas is famous for flash floods. One year, a wall of water came rushing through the creek bed in our yard and carried my animals away with it. Only two pairs of ducks survived, turning up a mile down the creek bed. I felt responsible and guilty. Perhaps I might have become a veterinarian, but this event was too painful. So I decided to be a Dr. Dolittle for people.

Heading East

When I finished high school the month after I turned sixteen, my parents were aware that I was still too immature, both socially and physically, to go to college. My father had gone to Princeton, where he'd been a star and had loved it, so I was destined to be sent there. My grades made the cut, but I was too small, too young and underdeveloped to be considered.

The question became where to send Berry to wait out his devel-opment. I felt like one of my animal specimens as they sized me up. Everyone in the two extended families was consulted. My uncle Charlie "Red" Eubank found me a place at his alma mater, Episco-pal High School in Alexandria, Virginia. EHS was a warm and friendly place where the children of elite southerners were sent to be prepared for southern colleges such as the University of Virginia or the University of North Carolina. A few went to places like Princeton. Since the emphasis at EHS was on scholarship, not pri-marily on athletics, it seemed right for me. And it was. I had a glo-rious, life-changing time during the two years I spent there.

From Waco to Washington, DC, was a two-day railroad ride. The day I left I stood on the platform at the end of the last car. All my Waco crowd came to see me off, then raced out to the next three or four crossings to wave at me en route. I wore a felt hat with the front brim turned down, hoping to look sophisticated and older. It was scary to leave home, but, by the first Christmas, I was hooked. At the constant holiday parties back in Waco, my hometown girlfriend and I clung together. Everyone said, "You've changed. You're already a Yankee!"

At EHS, all ages lived on wards of curtained cell-like roomettes with a bed and a shelf. Our lives were communal. This enforced closeness worked, but we had the typical adolescent cliques: the athletes hung out together, the preppies hung out together, the intellectuals hung out together. I found enough kids of my ilk to realize that I was not alone in my joy of learning. We read and shared ideas. I had a taste of feeling normal. Not the athletes my father might have wished for but kids who valued intellectual activities. I played enough tennis to "round me out," but my main pleasure and success at EHS was in my studies. I won several scholastic awards and was head of my class. I was even voted one of the most popular. What a turnaround.

Of course, my time at EHS was not completely blissful. One athletic star on my ward seemed to have it in for me. He teased me on every available occasion. "Teaberry, Gooseberry, Blackberry." He would slip down the hall at night after lights were out and crawl under my cot. There he lay, taunting me. In retrospect, it looks pretty sexually loaded, but I was too naïve to know that. He roused my anger and a desire for retaliation. I couldn't sleep after he slithered out. I wanted to "meet him behind the gym" but was too afraid of him. He was physically my superior, and I knew I had nothing to gain by confronting him. Unfortunately it reintroduced the doubts I'd already faced in Texas—that I was not an athlete or even able to defend myself. It brought back feelings of failing my father, his disappointment at my not sharing his passion for sports.

Princeton to Broadway?

Princeton University was—and is—apart from the real world. In 1938, there were no women, few—if any—minorities, and only a few Texans. For all of my four years there, I roomed with two classmates from EHS. We were not alike, not especially close, but we were a refuge for one another. We brought our southern heritage and our accents with us into Yankee territory. Of course I was intrigued by and jealous of all the wellborn Yankees. They hung out together and tolerated us but held us at arm's length. As a result, we southerners clung together for our social life as well. Later, when I branched out and got involved in theater and began to be accepted into the northern circles, my EHS friends felt deserted.

On weekends when I could afford to rattle up to New York on the Princeton shuttle, I was welcomed by Uncle Seth, Aunt Sing, and her daughter, whom we called Sister, who was just a little older than I. They lived in an elegant apartment on Park Avenue. Their way of life was a window into a sophistication and elegance I'd never known. Uncle Seth was chairman of the board of Standard Oil of New Jersey. Among other things they had lavish dinner parties—full of Russian royalty, princes and princesses who had fled from the revolution. Sister and I had whirls in the nightclubs of the city. I learned to love the glitz of New York.

Aside from the scholastics, Princeton taught me a great deal. I sang in the Glee Club. I rowed bravely but poorly on the freshman crew on Lake Nassau. I was asked to try out for and was accepted into the all-male Princeton Triangle Club. The Triangle was an esteemed organization that put on a musical every year. These productions involved Broadway directors of theatre (José Ferrer) and dance (Gene Kelly). Many luminous stars got their start here (Brooks Bowman, who composed "East of the Sun"; Joshua Logan, an important Broadway and Hollywood director and writer; and Jimmy Stewart). A Triangle musical would rehearse through the fall to build up to an East Coast tour during the Christmas holidays. We had a train with special cars we stayed in each night. Each city saved up its most special debutante party for our arrival. After all, here were seventy or eighty eligible, handsome Princeton men to flood the dance lines and to lap up their liquor and hospitality.

I found I could sing and dance. My first year, I was offered the male lead in *Any Moment Now* and sang my head off, stiffly, to all who'd listen. After the first year I played the female lead in three more shows, singing and dancing to applause. I could hardly believe it. In the various stops we made, I met with former Trianglers, including Jimmy Stewart, now successful in their post-Princeton years. I cavorted around in front of the chorus "girls" with hairy legs. After the show, real girls would flutter up to me. "How did you ever learn to be such a beautiful female?" "By watching you," I'd answer. I had "groupies" in every city, and my head became swollen. I was learning how to reach out for an audience and capture it. This experience has served me ever since. I never have any difficulty giving a lecture to a large audience.

I flourished at the Triangle Club, was elected president, and was wooed by the best eating clubs. I'd wanted to join Cap and Gown as my father had, but they wouldn't accept me with my three southern roommates. So I kept my allegiance to my fellow southerners, and we all joined the Charter Club. In spite of being from Texas, I was on the student council and had friends and even admirers. I was living in never-never land, a long way from Waco and from my childhood sense of inadequacy.

Meanwhile, I was pre-med and taking it seriously enough to have passing grades. I majored in chemistry, because I didn't have the foresight or the guts to try anything more dashing. I hated it. I tried to compensate by writing my senior thesis on sex hormones. That turned out to be a deadly and complicated subject, hardly related to my expectation of what I might learn about sex. I had to work very hard to pull out anything intelligible, but, when I finally did, my professor published it under his own name. He said he had worked on it too, but he hadn't. He gave me no credit at all. It was my first brush with the dirty politics of academia, but at least it got me graduated with good enough grades for medical school.

On a sad note, Bama died while I was at Princeton. I was twenty years old. I used to write to her from school and always went to visit her when I was home in Waco. I was still her favorite. I didn't get to see her before she died; I'd waited too long.

As I was about to graduate, Joshua Logan offered me an audition on Broadway. He said I could try out for the juvenile role with Ethel Merman in *Panama Hattie* and, if cast, play it all summer. If I wasn't successful during the summer run, then I'd go on to medical school in the fall. If I was successful, I could become a Broadway star. Jimmy Stewart even promised me a role in Hollywood movies. Excited, I called my parents in Texas. They were horrified. "Not only no, but hell no!" said my father. "Either you go to medical school and not be carried away by Broadway and Hollywood, or we wash our hands of supporting you!" In those days, one followed one's family's wishes. So, I turned down my one chance at Broadway. I've always wondered what it might have been like. However, I've managed to use my theater experience lecturing about children and families, and my twelve-year run on cable TV from 1984 to 1996 with *What Every Baby Knows* was all the more successful because of it.

TWO

Galveston to Boston:
Pediatrics and Psychiatry

After I finished Princeton, my father wanted me to be a Texan again. Although I had been accepted at Harvard, Columbia, and Johns Hopkins medical schools, he was certain that I'd never live in Texas if I stayed on the East Coast for medical school. So I went back, to the University of Texas medical school in Galveston.

Overall, I found medical school in Galveston boring, with the exception of anatomy. Grouped in fours, we were given cadavers. The first day, we all walked into the formaldehyde-permeated room with covered corpses scattered around, then into the adjoining lecture hall, dizzy from the smells and terrified of the imminent dissections. The cadaver for our group, which turned out to be that of the aunt of one of my classmates, had been found floating in Galveston Harbor. You can imagine how horrified he was as we tossed her organs at him during the dissection. Sadism had quickly become part of our first-year experience.

During my year in Galveston, I was asked to a festival every weekend—the Rose Festival in Tyler, a Mexican festival in San Antonio, the Cotton Palace in Waco, just to name a few. My social schedule quickly filled the time I should have been studying. Boredom was replaced with gaiety and pretty Texas girls. But I was not happy. I blamed it on having been pulled away from the East Coast. I knew I'd never get to be a good doctor if I stayed in Galveston. I wanted to be a doctor, not a socialite.

During the summer following my first year at Galveston, I went home to Waco. One Sunday, as was our routine, Mother and I went to church, leaving my father in his rocking chair reading. Church lasted its usual forever. When we returned home, we went upstairs to find my father dead in his chair. At the age of 49, in apparently excellent physical shape, he had suffered an overwhelming coronary. We never found out for sure, as no autopsy was performed. It was devastating. I felt that I should have known enough medicine to have predicted it or to have saved him by my far-too-late CPR methods when we found him. Mother was suddenly a widow. Chuck was still at Princeton. I thought that I'd returned to Texas in order to get to know my father better. We had both looked forward to knowing each other as adults, but it never really happened. I still get a feeling of something being unfinished. I've tried to make up for my inability to save him by filling every moment usefully.

After my father died, my uncle Charles took over the family business. Regrettably, Uncle Charles was a playboy, not a businessman and he drank up the capital of the Brazelton Lumber Company. Although we'd had an affluent life before, that was over. Mother had to go to work for the first time in her life, taking a job at Hill Printing Company selling stationery. I had to look for a scholarship in order to finish medical school.

Now that my father was gone, however, I could return to the East Coast. Mother was too grief stricken to argue. So, when Columbia University's College of Physicians and Surgeons offered me a scholarship, I was eager to snap it up and she agreed. I will never forget the elation I felt about going back East. During that summer, I had a chance to help my mother adjust to her new life, alone and in relative poverty. Though she was surrounded by her four sisters and many friends, she was a too-young widow. She rebounded and became an active and dedicated member of the Waco community, serving on the school board, starting a USO for the young soldiers who were stationed around central Texas preparing to go overseas. She also founded the first women's clinic in Texas that helped young women decide about terminating pregnancies. She was the first woman to become an elder at the Southern Presbyterian Church. But beloved as she was in Waco, Mother never had another relationship until she died in 1976.

Medical School—New York

To supplement my scholarship, I sold blood as often as I could and waited on tables daily. I lived in the dormitory at P&S, and because of my scholarship, I had no rent to pay. My mother sent me twenty-five dollars a month, which I took, but guiltily. I found ways to make my meager funds stretch far enough to include a social life.

Medical school in New York City was again a disappointment. Because I didn't arrive until second semester, others had already formed their cliques and support groups so it was hard for me to feel part of it. I felt brainwashed by the lecture system. There was no participation from us; there was no attempt to discuss clinical issues, and especially no help understanding the relationships with our patients. In sum, there was no real connection with any of the idealistic goals I'd hoped to reach by attending medical school. It was all hard science: pathology, histology, biology, and chemistry. Nothing about people. Later in my life, I watched as my son Tom went through a similar experience. Relationships with the patient and genuine care were scrapped in the service of disease and failing systems. I didn't learn much, I didn't perform well, and I don't remember much of it. Many years later, when I was awarded an honorary membership in AOA (the Phi Beta Kappa of medicine), I had to write to P&S for my record. They wrote back that no one had ever made AOA with such poor grades! Eleven honorary doctorates and an award for the most valued clinician of the P&S alumni later, I can grin inwardly. In my estimation, medical school does not fully prepare you for success in medical practice. That needs to be learned as you go. Ever since, I've wanted to change the training of young pediatricians to include more clinical experience and a knowledge of child development.

One professor, however, stood out. Professor of Medicine Dr. Robert Loeb, would have us stand at the end of the bed of a patient for fifteen minutes. We were to just observe and listen. At the end of that time after watching the patient, and without asking questions, we were asked to tell how old the patient was. We were asked what he did for a living, whether he was married or had children, what he was hospitalized for, and whether he was recovering. The amazing thing was that if you had watched the patient and listened to him or her carefully, you could answer all of these questions. I couldn't believe that observation could teach you so much. In my work as a clinician, I have used no other more useful technique. No other course in medical school was as rewarding, and I barely remember any of the rest of them.

Internship and WWII

When the Japanese bombed Pearl Harbor and the United States entered the war, we were rushed through medical school. As our peers were being sent to Europe and the Pacific, we were protected from the draft but were eager to do our part as physicians. It never occurred to me then, as it has since, to become a conscientious objector. In 1943, I volunteered for the navy.

Meanwhile I was very relieved finally to become an MD and assume my internship at Roosevelt Hospital in New York. I'd applied for internships all over New York City, but my grades and performance in medical school were pretty poor. I was lucky that Roosevelt was willing to take me.

All of a sudden medicine was on a par with my social life as the internship began to be fulfilling, and I found myself learning how to be a good doctor. Relationships and a critical eye turned out to be my forte. I became attached to my patients and they to me. I still hear from several families that I got to know as an intern in 1944. I'm still not sure how much medicine I learned as their doctor, but it was a wonderful, packed year of learning to be a clinician. I rode in the ambulances, delivered babies, went to Rikers Island prison, and patched up many tragedies. The year at Roosevelt Hospital taught me about life in a stressed, alcoholic, drug-filled part of New York. It taught me to handle emergencies, to deal with my own stress so I could reach out to others. I was drawn to younger patients and already realizing that I wanted to be a pediatrician, not an adult doctor.

In 1944, I was asked to report to the navy. I didn't know where my duties would take me. There was the Atlantic war and the Pacific war. The choice was up to the navy. Though I'd had one year of exposure to the acute and chronic problems of the inner city, I was still a baby, an inexperienced, raw graduate of medical school. I knew I was not prepared for what I was sent to do. I was scared, but everyone else was, too. Chuck was in France in the army with General Eisenhower. Everyone I knew was serving their country. All of a sudden, our relatively comfortable berths in hospitals were things of the past. With a two-continent war, the services needed as many of us as medical schools could provide. Our internships were cut short. Mine had been in medicine, with no surgery or exposure to trauma—the anticipated consequences of war. I felt very ill prepared. But who is prepared for war?

Shaking, I went to the Brooklyn Navy Yard in my fancy lieutenant junior grade uniform to learn of my assignment. I was to be the only doctor for 6 DEs (Destroyer Escorts—small ships designed to protect) accompanying ninety ships carrying supplies to Europe for the Allies, assigned to the USS *Dale Peterson*. These groups of ninety cargo ships crossed the Atlantic in ten days with six DEs protecting their assigned "herds" from the German submarines. The submarines were eminently successful in torpedoing these convoys and were slowing the progress toward victory by depriving Europe and our troops of necessary supplies. Our little DEs (half the size of regular destroyers) pitched sixty degrees from side to side in the rough Atlantic as they rounded the slower ships, using depth sonar to identify approaching submarines. When sonar found a sub, we would barrage them with depth charges to try to sink them before their torpedoes could be aimed at us. We torpedoed many whales but only one German sub in the Irish Sea. The crossings were dangerous but critical.

Living on one of these pitching vessels was a trick all its own. You never stopped propping yourself up. During the daytime you held on. During the nighttime you wedged yourself in a bunk to keep from being thrown out onto the steel floor. It was ten days per crossing each way from Brooklyn to London. Ten days was a long, long time. Fortunately, I have never been seasick, but the ship-mates who were paid a terrible price. One of our most important sonar experts, a chief sonar technician, lost ten to fifteen pounds on each crossing. He'd get to England, rehydrate and build himself back up in the three days' layover and then return to lose it all again on the return trip. His health and well-being was critical, as sonar was what protected all of us.

Medications never helped him. Finally, I found an ulcer diet that worked. I made him start drinking sugary, salty liquids every hour a day before we left and he was to continue them hourly all along. It worked and he continued to work our sonar and to pro-tect us.

Surgery at Sea

About three days into one trip to England, a corpsman on our ship developed an acute appendicitis. I knew I would have to operate on him. I'd never even seen an appendectomy in my medical training. I pulled out my copy of *Christopher's Surgery* and studied it intently, so frightened I could hardly read. I turned to the senior medical corpsman, an RN assigned to my ship. He said, "It'll be a breeze, I can help you. The biggest danger will be that either the patient or you will be thrown off the table by our forty-five to sixty degree rocking. Or your knife might slip." I was not reassured.

We set it up for two corpsmen to hold the patient on the table, another to hold me, and a fourth to turn pages of my book of sur-gery. The chief corpsman and I gave the patient a spinal anesthesia.

He was wide-awake during surgery and kept asking me, "What page you on now, Doc?" My knife didn't slip. I sweated profusely but one of the supporting corpsmen kept wiping my face. When we finally finished, the patient and I were both in shock. He recovered, but I didn't. He could even walk off the ship when we reached England. I barely could.

During that same crossing we blew up a Nazi submarine. Three German submariners floated to the top alive, their lower limbs already blighted with "immersion foot," a kind of circulatory failure brought on by being too long in the very cold water of the Irish Sea. Gangrene sets in and quickly becomes life threatening. I had to amputate the lower third of each gangrenous leg. Of course, I'd never seen an amputation. I got out *Christopher's Surgery* again. My chief corpsman and I went to work. Without him I'd have never managed. We amputated six legs. All of the Germans lived. Sixty years later, I still dream of those poor young men clomping around on the stumps I left them.

This was my contribution to World War II. Our ship's commander, Captain Bigelow, tried to get me awarded a medal for bravery. Needless to say, he didn't succeed. I wasn't that brave. I was responding to necessity.

At sea, I learned quickly to handle most things that occurred in the other ships by ship-to-ship phone. What I might have once felt necessary to see in order to make a diagnosis no longer seemed that urgent. I got very good at listening and diagnosing by telephone. This served me well when I got into pediatric practice later.

I recall the first time I had to make an actual ship-to-ship transfer. I had to be transferred via a breeches buoy. A breeches buoy is a wooden seat in the form of canvas "breeches" or pants hung from a life buoy suspended by ropes spanning from ship to ship. As long as the ships are rocking in synchrony, it's no problem, and the line can stay taut. But when they rock into each other, the line slackens and can get pulled into the propellers of one the DEs. I was certainly reluctant to try this procedure. But I had to. The two ships pulled alongside each other. They threw over the line, and I was helped into the swing. They were filming it as they transferred me, so I was able to watch this transfer later. The ships were synchronized—until I got halfway across. Then, all of a sudden they pitched into each other. The line dipped me into the water. I hung on to the ropes. Then, the ships pitched away from each other. My line snapped up, the swing threw me up into the air, and I flipped completely over the line. I continued to hang on. But I hit my head on the still line and began to sag in the seat, knocked out. I woke up just in time to grab the swing lines and complete the transfer. I have long since forgotten why I had to go over or whether the patient's illness was worth it, but I've never forgotten the trip. It taught me to wait to be sure I had to go over and to treat all I could by telephone.

When we arrived in England bringing ships loaded with supplies—food and ammunition both for the Allied forces and for an enormously stressed nation—we were welcomed as heroes. We did have our perks. Hermione Gingold, a comedienne who was the toast of the London theatre, took a fancy to me (and my gorgeous uniform). She sat me in a box next to the stage and played her comedy to me as I sat in the forefront of her audience.

When the war ended in 1945, I was given a choice to go to the Pacific and continue as a lieutenant junior grade in the navy, or to be discharged early. There wasn't a choice for me. I wanted out. Because I was discharged before others, I found there was less competition in the internship market. Hospitals everywhere were understaffed and hurting. As a surprising and happy result, I was accepted by Massachusetts General Hospital as a first-year pediatric intern.

Massachusetts General Hospital: A Focus on Pathology

Massachusetts General Hospital (MGH) was a web of buildings, so just learning how to get around was a year-long job. Although I was presumably welcome, there was no evidence of it when I arrived. No one seemed to speak to each other. If you asked directions to get around, people seemed to begrudge you the answers. Everyone was dour and unfriendly. When I spoke up with a suggestion for a case, someone would say, "Where did you learn that?" I would answer, "In New York at P&S." "Oh," they would say and that was the end of it. It took a big adjustment for me to get used to the Yankee reserve. But my patients' parents were delighted to find someone with a welcoming smile, and very quickly I had a raft of patients and people asking for me.

One night was I called to the Ringling Brothers train at North Station to see a baby with a 105-degree fever. The parents were the lead high-wire acrobats, and they were frantic about their year-old boy. When I arrived to see him in the train car, he was bright and perky in spite of his high fever. I found his "lovey," a baby doll, and he held it while I examined him. By then, I'd learned that no child likes to be descended upon until they know and trust you. I wanted to approach him gradually so I listened to each parent with my stethoscope. Then I placed it on the baby doll, then on the real baby. I made friends with him this way. His mother and father were grateful to see how easy he was with being examined. I found nothing to treat and told them so. Every night for three nights his temperature shot up to 104–5 degrees. During the day it was normal.

He never acted as if he were ill. When I examined him each evening, my anxiety rose but he reassured me by his behavior. I used no more special treatment except aspirin and liquids. (Today we never give aspirin to children for fever because it can cause serious side effects.) By the third night, I was able to promise the parents that his temperature would drop by the fourth day and that he'd get a pink scattered rash that looked like German measles but in reality was roseola. Roseola is a benign viral disease. It alarms parents, but it is a common disease in small children.

Because of the war, the hospital was terribly understaffed. We worked hard to make up for the inadequate coverage. We interns had to work two or three consecutive days around the clock. I learned to prop myself against a gurney and found I could sleep standing up. I could catnap and get by with twenty to thirty minutes' rest. We were really in crash mode. Many young doctors had not returned from the Pacific war, and MGH used this scarcity as a reason to hire fewer interns and residents than were really needed, in order to save money.

Pediatrics was chaired by a dynamic leader, Dr. Allan Butler. His brilliance kept us all on our toes. Many inquiring young MDs wanted to learn from him. Dr. Butler came to pediatrics from internal medicine, and he knew how to fight in the dog-eat-dog atmosphere of Harvard Medical School and MGH. He was a real radical and stood up, even at that time, for universal health care. Senator Joseph McCarthy, the witch hunter of that era, made him a target for his "communistic" views. I shared Butler's hopes and optimism and was intrigued that anyone believed we could really reach out to underprivileged people and change their lives. He advocated for AFDC (Aid to Families with Dependent Children) and health care that was subsidized, with systematic checkups and immunizations for every child. He believed in a preventive approach to pediatric care and warned that otherwise families would be left with only emergency medical care.

Thinking back, I see that he predicted our current medical situation more than a half century ahead. He believed that medical care would get fragmented and cost too much and that preventive care would not reach patients. His predictions have come true. Butler also started a study of the cost of providing free preventive health care for all the children of veterans who had gone to Harvard. It was called the Harvard Pediatric Study. After I began to practice pediatrics, I joined the study and learned so much from my association with the talented practicing pediatricians involved in it: Katherine Kiehl, Betty Gregory, Francis MacDonald. Butler wanted to find out whether free, preventive care could reduce or eliminate subsequent costs of hospitalizations if provided in a nurturing setting that reached out to all families. The study proved the benefits but, perhaps because of the political atmosphere at the time, was never published. Butler never got the honors he deserved.

My work at MGH was just as dreary as the atmosphere. I spent most of my time inserting tiny needles into the tiny veins of babies. Dr. Butler was developing electrolyte-containing fluids for intravenous use. Diarrhea indicated the need for intravenous fluids, so we were eager to admit any baby with diarrhea to the hospital. I remember one three-month-old we treated for twenty-eight days. A vein would wear out after three days and the line would have to be relocated. I used up all the available veins in this baby. She was still having liquid stools, so we felt justified in continuing her IV therapy. Finally, I found a tiny vein to one of her nipples. I got the needle in successfully and we continued her therapy. What it cost these babies and their parents for us to learn how to treat these dis-orders I cannot imagine.

I didn't feel comfortable with the kind of medicine being prac-ticed then at MGH, though I'm sure I learned a great deal about disease and pathology. Because MGH was *the* leading research cen-ter, it did encourage innovation.

To balance the clinical atmosphere of the hospital, I sought out friends. On a visit to Princeton, I met Edgar Romig, who had been in the class below me. His father was a Dutch Reformed clergyman. Edgar was teaching at Princeton Theological Seminary but his heart wasn't in it. I don't remember how he decided to come to Boston, but he ended up at Harvard Law School. Edgar and I roomed together in a little garret apartment, a fourth-floor walk-up, on Eaton Street (behind MGH) in an Italian neighborhood long since demolished. In our garret, we would play Puccini, eat pizza, drink cheap wine, and discuss the affairs of our respective worlds. Our friendship was very important to me. We added a third mem-ber to our group, a neophyte lawyer from Texas named Greer Tay-lor. Greer was brilliant and funny, and once a month he took us to the Ritz for dinner—"to touch the other world," he would say. These friendships and the fun we had together helped me balance the institutional chilliness at MGH and defend against the trag-edies of the sick children I saw.

For the most part, it was wonderful to treat children. Usually they were resilient and recovered from their illnesses, and all of the time they were responsive to a caring approach. But, when a child was seriously ill and couldn't recover, pediatrics was and still is a hellish profession. I've never built up enough of a shell. I still get very depressed when I care for a desperately ill child and his parents. It is hard for us as caregivers to face failures. At times our defenses against this may even make us seem insensitive.

Children's Hospital: Residency and Family

In 1948, I was asked to come to Children's Hospital in Boston for my last two years of residency. Although I had learned a great deal at Mass General, I hadn't learned to be a serious academic. I learned that at Children's.

There I was exposed to several pediatricians and fellow residents who were concerned with children's emotional development. All were interested in the "total child," not just their disease. It was a revelation to me. I was rotated through the House of the Good Samaritan, a special wing of the hospital where children with rheumatic fever were sent. At that time, children of all ages with rheumatic fever were put to bed for several years at a time if their fever went up to ninety-nine degrees every afternoon. It was a terrible disservice to growing children to be kept immobilized. Even though they were provided a schoolteacher from the Boston Public Schools, it delayed their development. They were depressed, hardly reachable, and emotionally a mess.

One nine-year-old got out of bed, climbed out a third-story window and literally crawled around the cement ledge. It seemed to me we were doing terrible things to these children in the interest of their medical recoveries. With two colleagues, Dr. Richmond Holder (a child psychiatrist) and Beatrice Talbot (a social worker) I wrote my first paper, "The Emotional Effects of Rheumatic Fever in Children," which was published in the pediatric literature of the time, the *Journal of Pediatrics*, 1953. With the advent of penicillin and its ability to master strep throats, the incidence of rheumatic fever went down dramatically. Because of this, we urged the House of the Good Samaritan to reconsider whether strict bed rest was necessary to the overall recovery of the children. It turned out that our paper spurred changes in the care of children with this chronic disease. No one had yet balanced the emotional cost to them with whatever minimal physical gains they might achieve by being kept in bed. Antibiotics have changed many of these practices, as has our attention to the balance between physical and emotional needs of developing children.

I loved my time at Children's Hospital. Compared to MGH, life was livelier and less depressing. I was amazed at the talents of my fellow residents. Many of them became professors of pediatrics— Bob Haggerty, Joel Alpert, Dane Prugh, Sam Katz, John Kennell, and many more. As residents at Children's in the years 1947–1949, we shared ideas in a way I had not been able to in any of my earlier medical experiences.

In 1949 my Texas friend and colleague Greer Taylor, who worked for Alfred Putnam Lowell, got me invited to the Lowells' house for a dinner party, and I was placed next to their third daughter, Christina. She was beautiful and very bright, but also very dignified and serious. She awed but frightened me. Months later, my friends Joe and Pat Edwards told me to ask her over for dinner with them at my Pinckney Street apartment. They overcame my hesitation and we asked her over. Smitten, I asked her if I could come to see her in New York City, where she worked at Putnam publishing company. She agreed. To bolster my chances, I took along a copy of an avant-garde poetry magazine with her cousin Robert Lowell's work in it. "Do you read this?" she asked. Of course I lied. She let me fall in love with her, and

I asked her to marry me that evening as our luncheon date was followed by a dinner date—lasting until 3:00 a.m. We were married in the fall of 1949—and have now passed our sixty-third anniversary!

Since my residency at Children's provided only $3,000 a year, I had to cut my hours there in half and start working at the Harvard Pediatric Study to make enough of a living to get married and support us. It was a fortunate choice, for I learned how to practice pediatrics and had a chance to try out my new psychiatric skills at a special clinic for children with mental health problems.

When Chrissy and I wanted to start a family, Mr. Lowell helped us buy a house in Cambridge. I was recruited by Dr. Ralph Ross, the leading pediatrician in Cambridge and set up a practice with him in Harvard Square. Chrissy was my secretary and helper until we began to make enough to hire one.

In 1951, our first daughter, Catherine Bowles, was born. She was so quiet and sensitive, such a contrast to many of my patients. The experience later led me to write my first book, *Infants and Mothers: Differences in Development*. I learned so much from each of my children.

Our second daughter, Pauline Battle (named for my mother) was born in 1954. She was feisty and fun and a contrast to her gentle sister. A third wonderful daughter, Christina Lowell Brazelton, was born in 1959. She was a beautiful baby and we thought we knew what we were doing as parents by then. Eight years later to our great surprise our son, Tom (Thomas Berry, III), came along and we were ecstatic.

At this time, my practice was booming, and we were beginning to be comfortably fixed in a wonderful Cambridge neighborhood. Chrissy was able to stay at home and be a mother for our four children. My career was taking off. I was able to teach, write, and practice and even do a half-time fellowship in cognitive development at Harvard with Jerome Bruner, a guru in developmental psychology (described in the next chapter). He opened the world of child development to me, and I was able to combine this knowledge and research with my pediatric and child psychiatry training. What lucky breaks!

Child Psychiatry

After my residency at Children's Hospital, I began to realize how little I still knew about children or their families. I needed to know more about their emotional lives. I recognized that mothers and children were on the defensive when they came into our hospital. They'd answer your questions in monosyllables. The child would either withdraw completely or start screaming. In our training, one learned how to keep a child on the table by holding him with one's own body. While he screamed away, you could then listen to his heart and lungs. I hated this kind of medicine. It was insensitive and controlling, telling parents how to raise their children (when we didn't know ourselves). I gradually got to know the parents of my patients and saw how they knew more than I did about their own child. Regrettably this thinking was not popular at the high-powered Children's Hospital.

When I finished my two years at Children's, our professor, Dr. Charles Janeway, called me to his office. He asked whether I'd be interested in taking on the job of running the outpatient department at Children's Hospital with Charles May, a well-known pediatrician. The job was a plum. Janeway was not only surprised but also chagrined when I told him I wanted to go into child psychiatry. I explained that I wanted to learn something about the relationships of children and parents. He disapproved, saying it was a "waste of good pediatric training!" I was disappointed by his lack of support for my choice. Later, when I had completed my psychiatric training and was back in pediatric practice, he sent his grandchildren to me. So I guess it wasn't such a terrible choice after all.

I divided psychiatric studies between the James Jackson Putnam Children's Center (founded by Marian Cabot Putnam in honor of her father) and Dr. Lucie Jessner at Mass. General's Department of Psychiatry. In doing so, I ventured out of my known field. Situated in an old house across from the Roxbury Latin School, the Putnam Center saw a real cross section of families and children. Then one of the most famous child psychiatric centers in the world, it was run by expert psychiatrists, many of whom had escaped the Nazis and had been welcomed in Boston. Among them were Myriam Davide from France; Dr. Beata "Tola" Rank, wife of one of Freud's pupils, Otto Rank; Eleanor Pavenstedt from Sweden; Dorothy MacNaughton from Scotland; and Eveoleen Rexford and Gregory Rochlin, two American child psychiatrists who practiced there. My contemporaries and fellow psychiatrists in training were Sam Kaplan and Gaston Blom.

I was the first pediatrician at the Putnam Center, and they hardly knew what to do with me. The first year they put me to work with Miriam Lasher, a talented child development psychologist. Miriam Lasher taught me a great deal, including how to get down on the floor and play with children. The next year, I learned to talk to parents under the tutelage of Harriet Robey, a social worker. She was my mentor and convinced me that psychoanalysis would solidify my psychiatric training. She helped me arrange to see a respected member of the Boston Psychoanalytic Society. At the consultation, I was stripped of my defenses. I unloaded all of my problems, my dreams and my hopes. At the end of the three-hour consultation, I literally shook with the revelations and the need to get going on an analysis. The analyst said, "Yes, I could help you. Make an appointment in two years." I was horrified. I couldn't find my car and even when I found it, I couldn't get the keys in the lock. I've never forgiven him for sending me out on my own after I'd exposed myself so thoroughly.

Back at the Putnam Center, I told this story to Harriet Robey and my psychiatrist friend Gregory Rochlin. Greg had also been a mentor while I was seeing children and their parents. He took pity on me and offered to take me on as an analysand right away. I had more than two rewarding years in analysis with him. Afterward, he became a friend as well as my former analyst. Today this would be a crossing of boundaries, but it was viewed somewhat differently back then.

During my third year at the Putnam Center, I was encouraged to practice as a child psychiatrist and to see patients. One of my patients was a four-year-old named "Skipper." Skipper was a skinny, blonde, and active but nonverbal child whose parents were overloaded by poverty, four other children, poor housing, too little to eat, and little hope of giving their five children all they wanted to give them. Skipper was assigned to me because his problems were not overwhelming. Though his parents knew he could speak, according to them he wouldn't. His mother was frightened, and she brought him to the Putnam Children's Center for therapy. Her priest joined in her concern and made her feel like a "failing mother." He urged her to seek help for Skipper "before it was too late." They thought he might have autism when he arrived at the Putnam Clinic.

With Greg Rochlin supervising, I felt safe in working with Skipper. He and I got along from the start. He was a kind and generous little boy. He shared toys with the other children in the playroom and comforted them when they cried by patting and stroking their cheeks. But he wouldn't speak. I could find no other defect in Skipper's makeup to call neurotic and leaned toward discounting his mother's plea for help. Skipper climbed up into my lap easily, and we played floor games without a hitch. But no words. "Skipper's trust in you is just beginning," Rochlin said. "Never underestimate a parent's cry for help." I thought Rochlin was crazy.

One morning, I was on the floor, playing with the other children in the room. All of a sudden, I felt warmth on my right shoulder. I reached up to find that my clothing was quite wet. Skipper had peed on my shoulder.

I was horrified but recovered enough to say, "Skipper, that's the first thing you've ever said to me. Thank you." Skipper looked surprised. He settled in my lap, reached up for my face, felt my mouth and began to speak. He called me "Papa." Our therapy began, and, within a few months, he was speaking and relating to his parents and siblings with ease. It was my first success in child psychiatry— thanks to his knowing how to reach me.

Meanwhile, Lucie Jessner at MGH had given me a much more difficult case to treat. Though she mentored me, I was essentially in charge. The case involved a withdrawn fourteen-year-old Jewish girl from Worcester, Massachusetts, who had been at Children's Hospital before she was transferred to MGH. We learned that her older sister had confided in her that she'd had sexual relations, was pregnant, and planned to marry a Gentile. Her parents were completely against it, and the girl, whom I'll call "Anne," was caught in the middle. She developed hysterical symptoms. She wouldn't walk and just lay in bed, presumably helpless.

At Children's Hospital, in order to prove that Anne was "faking," her attending neurologist got her on her feet and made her walk for the medical students. She withdrew completely after this exposure—wouldn't eat, drink, void, or move her bowels and was transferred to the psychiatric division at MGH. Lucie Jessner asked me to become her therapist because I was also a pediatrician and could supervise her physical management. Everyone was terrified of her not drinking, eating, voiding or moving her bowels. They wanted to implant a feeding tube, an intravenous line to hydrate her, and a catheter to void her urine. I felt she'd been so mishandled already by medical people that I wanted to try to treat her hysteria without invasive methods. Some thought I was crazy, but I wanted to see whether she and I could accomplish her recovery together with a psychiatric approach. I instructed the nurses not to push her to eat or drink. They could leave a glass of water at her bedside but put no pressure on her to drink it. There would be no catheter, no suppositories, and no other medical interventions. I saw Anne two or three times a day in order to establish a relationship with her that she could trust. I hoped that then she might share her problems with me. Every day, the nurses and doctors would ask me, "Shouldn't you act now, Brazelton?" "Doesn't she need an IV or a catheter or a laxative?" But I'd set out on a course, and I wanted to stay with it.

One evening, the nurses called me out of a party to tell me that she'd snuck a bit of water. What a triumph! She began to sneak water and juice daily, on the fifteenth day, she urinated spontaneously, and, finally by the twentieth day, she ate her first solid food. Her bowels began to move, and by the end of the month, she was recovering physically and we began to be able to talk about all that she'd been through.

I continued to see her for another year and a half. She recovered completely after treatment for the weakness in her legs caused by being bedridden for so long. Later, she got her college degree, married, and had two children. I believed then as I do now that Anne's progress toward recovery showed how powerful combining pediatrics and psychiatry can be.

THREE

Discovering the Power of Newborns

In the early 1950s it was still assumed by many that newborn babies were "lumps of clay," ready to be shaped by their environment. Hence, any deviation in their development, mild or severe, even autism, was blamed on the parents. At the James Jackson Putnam Children's Center where I worked at the time, parents who brought their infants for assessment and therapy were therefore themselves often seen in psychotherapy. But the parental therapy did not enhance the baby's progress, and the expectation that it was needed to make them better parents only increased their suffering. Babies on the autism spectrum, for instance, are difficult to reach no matter how hard their parents try. When the babies we cared for had brain damage and delayed development, their progress was slow and their outcomes not optimal, despite parents' desperate efforts. Premature infants, too, were slow to catch up, and therapy with their parents did not seem to help their development. Nevertheless, parents were still being blamed and were ready to be blamed. They were treated with psychotherapy year after year, but their babies did only marginally better.

The Baby's Contribution

I began to feel that we were missing the point. All of these babies presented challenges for their parents that were not their parents' fault, and blaming them was counterproductive. It seemed like blaming the victim. Parents are already vulnerable to being blamed; they feel responsible for any defect or problem. Their feeling of guilt comes from caring deeply. As a pediatrician observing the ways these babies were hard to reach, I could see that what parents needed was support in their difficult task. Allowing the parents to become immobilized with guilt made them less able to work toward the infant's recovery. If we could evaluate these infants as newborns and share our understanding with parents, I thought we could help them bring out the potential in their babies. The baby's contribution to the relationship was not recognized. Parents who were aware of this contribution could work with us to help their particular baby progress. Otherwise, these vulnerable parents just withdrew and became defensive and couldn't be reached. Sometimes, they later abused or neglected their difficult babies.

Although competent assessments of a newborn's neurological status had been developed by Heinz Prechtl, a neuropsychologist in Holland, they did not include the babies' sensory responses or their ability to respond to parents' nurturing attempts. The feedback systems between a newborn baby and a passionate parent could be enhanced by our understanding of how each baby functioned. If we could evaluate a baby's ability to adapt to a parent's efforts, we could help parents tailor their efforts to the baby's needs from the first. By evaluating newborns as early as possible, we could design therapeutic approaches from which infants at risk for various reasons (premature, small for gestational age [SGA], etc.) could profit from the beginning.

My growing pediatric practice made me aware that many of the children who showed delays in development had unusual behavior from the first. Many babies had erratic responses and were hard to reach. A baby on the autism spectrum was often unable to respond to parents' interactions and avoided visual contact. Some of the other infants we treated at the Putnam Center had other sensory or physical problems that contributed to their difficulties from the first. If I could devise ways to evaluate newborn responses, I thought I could help predict the kinds of difficulties that an individual baby would present to parents.

In studying these earliest relationships, I was helped by the fine work of Stella Chess and Alexander Thomas, who introduced the concept of differences in children's temperaments. These differences were initially genetic, but they affected the parent-child interaction in ways that could interfere with development. Sybille Escalona had also written about differences such as thresholds of hyper- and hypo-sensitivity in infants. I saw that understanding these findings and sharing them with parents could enhance their future together.

Finding a Baby's Best Performance

Well before all this research, parents already knew their newborns were responsive to lights and sounds in the uterus. After birth, they could see the responses for themselves. However, most pediatricians, developmental psychologists, and neurologists hadn't accepted these observations. They were blinded to the full range of babies' responses by a flaw in the way they tested them. To test sensory modalities in newborns, experts undressed them, laid them out on a table, and presented them with lights and sounds. The babies reacted only sporadically because they were protecting themselves from these intrusive sensations by "habituating," or shutting out the sensations. They might have shown reliable responses had the examiners brought them gently to a comfortable, alert state. As a result, no one would accept that newborns were really seeing or hearing. Parents' observations were not taken seriously.

Elsa Peterson, a neonatal nurse at the Boston Lying-In Hospital with many years of experience, gave me my first insight into the effort a stressed baby must make to respond. She and I (then a pediatric resident) were watching two very immature, sick preemies as they gasped for breath in their incubators. Elsa said, "Watch that one, she'll be breathing OK in three more days, but the other one will take six or seven more days." She was always right, so I said, "How do you know?" She replied, "Watch the first one. She can stop breathing briefly as she looks up at the light over her crib or responds to the overhead lights or the noises in the nursery. Then, she'll go on breathing. Her lung development and heart controls allow her to adjust to brief signals [auditory and visual] from around her. The other one can't do that yet, but he will mature enough to be able to in another three or four days." And she was right. She was the first to point out to me the interaction between the physiological demands of babies' immature lungs and heart systems and their ability to control these systems in order to take in their new world. Even a preemie can see and hear, and, if it matters enough to her, she will try to control her breathing. But the demands of her lungs and her heart must come first, as they are necessary to her survival. Once those basic needs are met as she matures, she can become alert and respond to sights and sounds more easily.

At around this time, Lula Lubchenco, a neonatologist at the University of Colorado, had constructed a score of the risks at birth to a baby's well-being. She coupled this with a score to evaluate and predict the survival of fragile infants. Visual and hearing responses played a major role in her assessment. Among the initial risk factors were disturbed intrauterine experience and stressful delivery. Lubchenco then assessed the newborn's appearance, whether her development was appropriate for her date of birth or whether she was small for her gestational age. In addition, she looked to see how the baby was adjusting to birth, delivery, and her new environment. If she was able to respond to sounds, sight, and touch, Dr. Lubchenco felt she was in optimal shape and could be allowed to leave the neonatal intensive care unit (NICU) and go out to her mother or to a normal nursery environment. Such a baby, she predicted, could even be breast-fed right from the first and could avoid going to the NICU. Her scoring of risks and the baby's responsiveness was innovative and important because it helped make decisions about care. Her predictions were amazingly accurate and made a deep impression on me. No other investigator before her had considered the babies' ability to manage their autonomic systems after birth as a predictor of later well-being.

Sally Provence, a pediatrician at the Yale Child Study Center, also showed me how to bring out a newborn's rich responses. She loved newborns and believed in babies' competence. She knew that you needed to support and contain them so they could respond. She would swaddle a newborn baby, wrapping his arms and legs with a blanket, then hold him in her arms at a thirty-degree angle, which alerts a baby. She'd sway gently in a rhythm to help the baby come to an alert state. As she virtually danced with the baby, the baby would become more alert. She'd sing quietly, dance slowly, and the newborn baby would open his eyes and become responsive to her. The newborn would follow her voice and her face. Sally demonstrated vividly that the baby could not only see and hear but would respond when handled appropriately.

I found her work thrilling. "Sally, it looks like you get inside a baby's brain!" "Well, there's a baby inside each of us, isn't there?" In that sentence, she hinted at the underlying, unconscious reason each of us responds to a new baby. She confirmed for me how critical it was to contain the baby's random motor activity in order to help him go from a shutting-out state to one in which he was able to be alert and responsive. I began to realize why researchers hadn't been able to get reliable visual and auditory responses from newborn babies. They didn't account for the newborns' need to control both their autonomic and motor systems before becoming able to respond. Sally first helped the baby achieve state control, then he could respond to sensory stimuli. Others could then see these responses and believe in them.

Later on, I went to St. Louis to observe the work of Dr. Frances Graham. Her scale was the first to measure the baby's ability to respond visually. I also watched Bettye Caldwell (a psychologist) as she showed what she had to do for the baby to produce these visual responses. First, she swaddled the newborn. Then she gave her a pacifier "to get her energy up to her mouth." Then, she gradually withdrew the pacifier, slowly to avoid a protest, while presenting a red object that the newborn then fixed on with her eyes. She moved the ball back and forth, turning the baby to follow it, maintaining her alert state for several minutes at a time. In this way, Caldwell demonstrated that a baby's energy might be available to be manipulated. It was not yet a scientific observation, but the opportunity to watch a prominent psychologist encourage the visual capacity of the newborn and "move the energy from her mouth to her eyes" was exciting and spurred me on.

Developing the Neonatal Behavioral Assessment Scale

I began to look for ways to produce visual and auditory responses reliably and to develop a scale that measured these responses. Heinz Prechtl was famous for identifying neurological impairments in babies by deficits in their motor behavior (he could identify cerebral palsy and other motor disorders due to brain damage at an early stage). In seeking to distinguish which motor differences were due to brain disorders and which occurred just because the baby was asleep or not responsive to his tests, he found that the baby's state when tested was critical to the quality of her motor behavior. In constructing his scale, he identified six different states of consciousness (deep and light sleep, an indeterminate state, wide awake, fussing, and crying).

I began to see how useful the six states would be in examining babies, allowing them to use their control systems to achieve their best responses to sensory stimuli. These states were the matrix on which different kinds of newborns' responses depended. It all began to fall in place for me. Unless one respected the state of the baby, you couldn't get reliable responses. In alert states, motor or sensory responses could be optimal. In sleep or crying states, the baby would be less responsive to sensory stimuli or lose motor control. Gerald Stechler and I demonstrated that newborns alert to interesting stimuli and put themselves into a sleep state in order to avoid repeated negative, intrusive auditory or visual stimuli. We assessed newborn responses using electroencephalographic (EEG) leads on the infant's head, and we also had respiratory and heart rate recordings. When we presented babies with a very bright light, they startled. The first few lights continued to cause startles, EEG changes, and respiratory and heart rate changes. By the tenth or twelfth stimulus, however, the infant would stop responding. And by the fifteenth stimulus, he produced an EEG record that looked like deep sleep. He had simply put himself to sleep to shut out disturbing stimuli. When we stopped after twenty stimuli, he then awoke, thrashed around, and by fussing and crying discharged the energy it had cost to suppress these responses. What a powerful mechanism habituation was. It was absolutely necessary to any newborn in a noisy, overlit environment.

This was an entirely new idea at the time—habituation followed by the discharge of energy to recover the cost of suppressing responses to stimuli that would otherwise overwhelm and disorganize the baby. As a result of understanding this ability to adapt, we came to realize that a baby's central nervous system was able to avoid overloading the cardiorespiratory systems by shutting out sensory stimulation that was too demanding. Habituation seemed to resemble sleep on the EEG. A baby who couldn't shut out responses to stimuli would be at the mercy of his environment. Normally, a baby has the ability to control his brain's reactions to a loud sound, a bright light, or repeated intrusive stimulus of any kind—visual, auditory, tactile, or even kinesthetic. As he does so, one can observe his heart rate and breathing become regular and steady. As he moves into a state similar to deep sleep, he is "actively" shutting out all stimuli, and this costs him a good deal. But moving into deep sleep is not as costly as being responsive. He begins to breathe slowly and steadily, and his heart rate slows and becomes regular.

This is why, when neurologists or psychologists in the past unwrapped babies (exposing them to cold air) and laid them out on a table (without any protection from their own startles), they would not see the babies' range of responses. These were noxious stimuli that the baby needed to shut out. At least half the time, babies would go into a habituated state. This meant that they often looked as if they could not "see" or "hear." Not only are babies' movements very different in each state (as Prechtl had pointed out) but their responses to the efforts of others to reach them would be different.

I then worked to figure out how to produce the baby's optimal performance. I saw that a dressed, swaddled baby acted very differently from an undressed, unprotected one. I found that babies lying down flat on their backs and at the mercy of startles that they couldn't control would not be very responsive. Held at a thirty-degree angle, as Sally Provence showed, they would alert to a responsive state. As I played with newborns in the newborn nursery, I could get them to turn their heads, to follow my voice, my face, a red ball, or a soft rattle. And they'd work to stay under control, awake and responsive. When they became overwhelmed, they protected themselves with sleep, drowsiness, or crying. I began to see these abilities as a great strength. They were critical to newborns, attempting to learn about the world—from the first. As I found I was able to elicit these powerful abilities, I could hear my grandmother's voice: "Berry is so good with babies."

Building on these observations, I began to design a test that we called the Neonatal Behavioral Assessment Scale (NBAS). Using Prechtl's six states of consciousness as a base, we became successful in producing reliable sensory responses that were balanced with motor and autonomic responses. These responses, in turn, became a way of understanding the individuality and temperament of each baby.

A Newborn's Six States

Deep Sleep. The infant's eyes are firmly closed and still. There is little or no motor activity, with the exception of occasional startles or rhythmic mouthing. The baby's abdomen rises and falls with her breathing, which is relatively slow (an average of thirty-six breaths per minute), deep, and regular.

Light Sleep with Rapid Eye Movement (Dreaming). The infant's eyes are closed and under her lids eye movement (REM) can be seen. Activity can range from minor twitches to writhing and stretching. Breathing is irregular and generally faster than seen in deep sleep. The baby's expressions include frowns, grimaces, smiles, twitches, mouth movements, and even sucking. But she is not yet beginning to awake.

Drowsy State. The infant's eyes may open and close or may be partially open, but she appears dazed. She may move around a bit. Breathing is a bit faster and more shallow.

Alert Inactivity. Now the infant's body and face are quiet and under control, her eyes appear bright and shining, and she will follow a red ball or the examiner's face. She will turn toward a voice or any sound. This is the fun state for an examiner and for parents. It sometimes seems as if the baby is even attempting to maintain this state in order to interact with the examiner.

Fussing. Agitated vocalizations begin. The baby fusses and squirms. She won't follow or turn to a sound with interest like she did before. A few cries may break out.

Crying State. The whole body is moving, and the cry bursts are continuous. The baby's color changes, her skin reddening. Now she responds only to swaddling, holding, something to suck, or an intrusive voice or light. A look at the examiner's face can stop her between bursts, but she is likely to be unavailable to any but controlling measures—those of the examiner or her own, such as putting her hand to her mouth and sucking.

As soon as I began to play with babies using this concept of the control of states, it was like going under water for the first time with goggles and seeing all the fish one never saw before. Babies' behavior is so complex and exciting, if you provide the support they need.

For example, when a newborn is crying in her crib and you lean down next to her ear and talk steadily to her, she will stop after a short bit and look up into your face gratefully. She has used your voice to help herself gain control. Or put a newborn up on your shoulder to cuddle her. Soon she will pick up her head, look around the room, mouth her fist, then nestle her soft little scalp into the corner of your neck. With a sleepy baby, hold her at a thirty-degree angle looking in your face. If you need to, rock her a bit to awaken her. As soon as she sees your face, her own will alert as if she were ready to smile and vocalize at you. She wants you to talk to her softly in this alert state.

When you place a baby on the diaper table, holding her firmly, and talking while cleaning her, she'll look quietly and gratefully at you, ready to smile or vocalize. She will quickly learn that this is a time for communication. A newborn's responses are so thrilling. Whenever I'm with a newborn, I feel the magic in the way each baby plays a role in furthering the relationship with those who care for her and, as a result, her future.

The reflex system is another important element in assessing a newborn's intactness. Certain reflexes at birth are signs of a normal nervous system, assuring us that the baby is not brain damaged. These include (1) the walk reflex (which will go underground over the next few months, to return as voluntary walking), (2) attempting to hold her head up as she is pulled up by her arms to sit, (3) picking her head up when she is laid face down and turning her head to free her airway, (4) rooting: when either cheek is stroked, her head will turn to try to grab the stroking finger with her mouth, (5) sucking on anything—a finger, the breast, the bottle, or a pacifier, (6) bringing her hand to her mouth to comfort herself, (7) startling when she is handled abruptly, (8) grasping a finger or other object held out to her, (9) the tonic neck reflex—when the baby's head is turned to one side, the body arches and the arms come into a fencing position, and (10) the gallant reflex, in which the baby is held face down and stroked on one side of the spine. The baby moves her hips toward the stroked side. This last reflex helps a baby squirm her way out of the uterus.

By paying attention to the states of a baby, an experienced examiner can make a fairly accurate prediction of how a baby will respond to any given stimulus. For example, within a deep sleep state, a baby responds only slightly to a moderate rattle; although breathing changes and blinking may occur, the child probably stirs or rouses very little. As she changes to a light sleep state, slower movement of the arms and legs begin, and her trunk will writhe as she awakens to the stimulus. The baby will open her eyes to look around dully. In the semialert state, the baby begins to move about and will even search for stimulus. When she reacts to a soft rattle or a voice, her breathing becomes slower and more regular. She moves to a wide-awake state in which she can pay attention. Her face and body become quiet. She looks surprised and turns to follow the sound. Her head turns, her body remains still as she follows the sound from side to side. Some newborns can maintain the alert state for quite a while before they begin to tire and start to fuss as they retreat into sleep.

The NBAS and the New Parent

As we developed the scale, often called the Brazelton scale, we began to see that sharing the baby's individual responses at birth was a powerful way of preparing new parents for their role. In numerous published papers, I and other researchers documented the value of sharing with new parents a professional assessment of their newborn's powerful abilities. This gives parents a vivid insight into their own individual baby.

Parents are bound to be captured by this array of behavior. They will work very hard to understand their baby and to produce not only responses but to bring out the baby's "best performance" as they handle her. When a baby turns to her mother's or father's voice, the parent feels "She knows me!"

Thus, not only could the scale be a way of assessing the baby's contribution to the parent-infant relationship but also the parent's responses gave a window into the level of sensitivity they brought to their baby. As I worked with the scale, I felt it could predict the nature of the parent-infant's future attachment.

Understanding the nature of the sleep state is also helpful to parents. When a baby moves from deep to light sleep, she will rouse, cry out and thrash around, as if she were discharging stored up energy, before she can drop back into the more protected state of deep sleep. In nighttime sleep, these states oscillate every ninety seconds, but the baby appears to remain in what seems to be deep sleep until she comes up to the light sleep state every three to four hours. Then, she will rouse and discharge motor activity and her heart rate and breathing become jerky and irregular. In light sleep she is available to external stimuli and will wake up if stimuli are presented to her. Parents need to see how hard she works to protect herself in deep sleep and how available she is to rouse from light sleep to an alert, responsive state. When it is not the middle of the night, parents may find the light sleep state a time to begin to play with her, to learn more about her.

In working with the NBAS, I saw how exciting it was to caregivers and parents to notice that as a baby follows the human face, she becomes even more actively engaged than she does with an object. If the examiner speaks as well as presenting her face, the baby's features become mobile. Meanwhile, her motor activity and even her heart rate seem to be controlled so that she can pay attention. After a while, when she shuts off or changes to a fussy or a crying state, the baby shows how much this interaction costs her immature nervous system. She is liable to be exhausted, to drop into a sleep state and become unavailable. It helps parents to know that a baby needs to recover before she can interact again.

Parents of fragile babies need to learn the signals that indicate a baby is overwhelmed—yawning, hiccoughing, frowning, spitting up, or having a bowel movement. Eyes rolled up and away, arching, or a flaccid body can also be signs of "I've had enough." A new parent begins to learn this language of self-protection. The baby seems to be saying, "I want to interact and learn about you and my new world—as long as I can." But when her system is overloaded, she seems to say, "I've had enough. Give me time."

A parent also learns the difference between cries (hunger, pain, fatigue, discomfort, overstimulation), and then learns what to do about them. Crying is a powerful communication between the baby and the parent. All parents want to learn to tell the differences.

Parents often said to me, "I wish someone had sent me home with a book about how to care for this baby." My answer was: Well, they have. Your baby will tell you what works for her and what doesn't. Just follow her responses and behavior and you'll learn how to become a parent for her. You'll learn more from your mistakes than from your successes. When you try something and it doesn't work you'll try six or seven other ways to reach her. When one finally works, you'll have learned from all these seven or eight tries.

Refining the Scale

In addition to proving the competency of babies and showing that deviations are not a parent's fault, the goal for the NBAS was to record the responses within each state—autonomic, motor, sensory—that integrated with each other in the normal, healthy, full-term infant. The NBAS was not meant to be a set of discrete stimulus-response presentations but an interactive assessment of the performance and self-organizing skills of the infant. We hoped to establish the infant's contributions to the caregiving environment. Repeated examinations demonstrated the infant's ability to use his inner organization to experience and profit developmentally from environmental stimulation. The infant's use of different states to maintain control of his reactions to environmental and internal stimuli reflects his potential for organization. We demonstrated that changes in states no longer needed to be treated as a hindrance to assessment. Instead, by respecting states we could see the infant's full behavioral repertoire. The NBAS tracks changes in state over the course of the examination and the direction of these changes. The variability of states, both the infant's ability to quiet himself and his search for stimulation, reveal his capacity for self-organization.

The NBAS came to include eighteen reflex measures and twenty-eight behavioral responses to environmental stimuli, including the kind of interpersonal stimuli that mothers and fathers use in handling

their infants. In the examination, there is one graded series of procedures (e.g., talking, hand on belly, restraint, rocking) designed to
soothe the infant and another to arouse him. His responsiveness
to animate stimuli (e.g., voice, face) and to inanimate stimuli (e.g.,
rattle, bell, red ball, white light, temperature change) is assessed. Esti-
mates of vigor and attentional excitement are measured, and an
assessment is made of motor activity, tone, and autonomic responsiveness as the infant changes state. Supplementary items to rate
other observations have been added, such as cost to the neonate of
the assessment, level of effort required of the examiner to elicit the
infant's best performance, and the quality of his best performance.
These additional questions ("How hard did you have to work to
get the baby's best performance?" and "Would you take this baby
home?") helped us identify the nature of the parents' job as they tried
to relate to their baby. The answers to these questions were amazingly
predictive. Developmental psychologist Marjorie Beeghly assessed
children at the age of three and found that these answers were still
descriptive of the child's performance and temperament. This seemed
a testimony to the infant's individual differences in the newborn
period, as well as to the infant's strong influence in shaping parents'
nurturing.

Tiffany Field, the first person trained in the NBAS, has been a
major contributor to research in infancy and in parent-infant communication. A prodigious researcher, she often confirmed the different uses of my NBAS with her research paradigms. Tiffany
developed the importance of touch as a form of parent-infant communication, including massage. Different kinds of touch denoted
different messages. A light touch might mean, "Hello, I'm here.
Can you respond to me?" A heavier touch might mean reassurance.
An even heavier touch could be used to help a baby gain control.

Each different kind of touch might set the state for a different response from the infant.

By performing the NBAS on successive days, we were able to outline a newborn's recovery from birth: the initial period of alertness immediately after delivery, the period of depression and disorganization that follows, and the curve of recovery after several days. The period of depression and disorganization lasts twenty-four to forty-eight hours in infants with uncomplicated deliveries and no medication effects, but it persists for three to four days in infants slowed by medications given during delivery. The curve of recovery may be an early predictor of individual potential and seems to correlate well with the neonate's abilities when tested thirty days later.

My peers in infant research had several criticisms of the scale: (1) only Brazelton knows what "best performance" is, (2) it can't be reliable from one observer to the next, and (3), it doesn't predict to the baby's future. All of these criticisms we took seriously. To answer the first two we began to increase our requirements for reliable training—so stringently that we may have scared away most clinicians. Researchers, however, have welcomed it, and nearly a thousand papers have been published on the scale by reliably trained observers. To test the prediction, we have used three consecutive assessments over the first month—at birth, at two weeks, and at four weeks, including all the behavioral responses as well as the reflex behaviors. Apart from the recovery after medication at birth, assessments that improve over the month demonstrate the infant's ability to incorporate nurturing from his environment. The responses and behaviors that don't change are probably genetic and fixed in the newborn period. The responses that are changing, but not in a positive way, are those that deserve our attention. Concerning children with special needs, these assessments can provide us with guidance for an early intervention program to help infants live up to their underlying potential. We learned how powerful these distinctions are by using the scale with premature and high-risk infants.

The work with premature infants led Barry Lester, Ed Tronick, Heidi Als, and me to develop the APIB (Assessment of Premature Infant Behavior). It is a very detailed assessment of premature, fragile infants and is now widely used. With it, Heidi Als has been able to demonstrate that changing NICU nurseries to respect the fragile, easily overloaded nervous systems of immature babies makes a significant difference in their outcomes. By reducing noise, light, and painful, disturbing handling, these babies not only recover much more quickly, but they incur significantly fewer ophthalmic difficulties, respiratory problems, and gastrointestinal complications. Heidi's creative application of the scale significantly improved these babies' futures, and she calls this new kind of care developmental care. She has developed a methodical process called the Newborn Individualized Developmental Care and Assessment Program for NICUs to use as they bring about this transformation.

While developing the APIB, we also learned a great deal about parents' adaptation to a premature birth. Even when parents appear to recover from their expectable grief about their baby's prematurity or high risk, we still need to do more work to help them relate to the baby. I have identified four stages that parents must go through in order to be ready to attach to their fragile baby: (1) speaking of the baby as if she were just chemicals (pH, O_2, electrolytes, etc.) being measured by the apparatus of the NICU, (2) seeing that the baby responds with reflexes to a medical person (nurse or doctor), (3) seeing that the baby responds to others with behavioral responses (turning to their voices, alerting when another person comes up to the crib), and (4) expecting the baby to respond to the parents themselves with such behavior. We have found that in addition to Als's work to change the NICU, the outcome of premature infants was improved if we encouraged the parents through these four stages of recovery. The nurses can monitor this progress; for instance, their notes might say "Mother is in stage 4, but father is in stage 2. Work on father." With support, parents of premature infants become ready to attach to them before they are discharged, and their future relationships are improved.

Troublemaking in the Delivery Room

Because I was so interested in newborns, I came to care how they were delivered, how much premedication their mothers received, and how a long labor affected them. One of my first papers on newborn behavior compared babies who were delivered without premedication to babies whose mothers had received the then routine "twilight sleep" (an opiate, usually morphine, used with scopolamine) for labor. There was already a great interest in "natural childbirth," including techniques pioneered by Dr. Fernand Lamaze, a French obstetrician. He educated mothers about labor and delivery and, by supporting them during labor, was successfully delivering babies in France without medication. My study showed that newborns whose mothers had been premedicated two to twelve hours before birth had slower deliveries. At birth they had good Apgar scores (Apgars reflect the baby's response to labor and delivery), which showed that these newborns could rouse adequately to the stress of labor and delivery. Thirty to sixty minutes later in the newborn nursery, however, they began to struggle. Nurses spent their time helping these newborns cough up thick mucus. Babies are born ready to cough up mucus and amniotic fluid in their airways, so that their lungs can start absorbing air, but if they are too sedated and difficult to rouse, they don't respond enough to stimulation and don't cough up the mucus without help. An unmedicated infant can cough it up easily and without help.

As soon as the cord is cut, the baby's level of sedation is set. The medication mothers had received is stored in the newborn, affects her immature brain, and is slowly excreted by her immature kidneys or slowly detoxified by her immature liver. The babies of medicated mothers showed a diminished responsiveness for seven to ten days after delivery. Their mothers had difficulty in rousing them for breastfeeding. Thus, it was hard for parents to see their baby as a responsive person for the first week.

My opinions on this matter became known. I remember walking down the halls of the Boston Lying-In Hospital one day when I heard a resounding command, "Dr. Brazelton, come here!" It was Dr. Duncan Reid, professor of obstetrics at Harvard Medical School and head of the Lying-In. "That study you did on the effects of medicating mothers is ruining my whole career!" He went on to say that he'd worked for forty years to develop medication to ease labor for suffering mothers. He found their labor excruciating to watch and wanted to make it easier for them. But there was a cost. My paper helped lead a re-evaluation of maternal premedication and its effects on newborn babies. At that time a number of groups around the country were trying to naturalize and demedicalize birth. Dr. Marshall Klaus from Case Western Reserve medical school in Cleveland was a leader in this effort. He and his colleague, my friend then at Children's Hospital in Boston, Dr. John Kennell, had written papers on how important it was for babies to be alert and responsive so that parents could bond with them right after birth. They were the first advocates of attachment between mothers and babies. They described bonding and how it became passionate, starting from the immediate period after birth. Their important work has unfortunately been misunderstood and taken too literally. Some mothers needlessly worry that they can never make up for this first great period of bonding if something, like a medical emergency, prevented it.

Marshall and I were asked to lecture all over the country to further the movement for natural childbirth. One night I said to Marshall, "I can't stand to give this lecture in front of you one more time." He replied, "I can't stand to hear it again. I'll tell you what: you give my lecture, and I'll give yours." We did, and it was fun! A good way to deal with burnout. I think our efforts made a real difference. Hospitals all over the country began to buy into natural childbirth, Lamaze, and other techniques.

I witnessed one of the first attempts at the Boston Lying-In Hospital to use these techniques. Dr. Arthur Gorbach (a young, brave, and forward-looking obstetrician) was delivering a baby. A midwife and the father were supporting the mother through the labor. One of the suggestions was to keep the labor room quiet and darkened, so the mother wouldn't be distracted and could concentrate on her labor. Dr. Gorbach would issue a loud "shush" every time anyone made a sound (except the mother-to-be, of course). When the baby finally came and let out a few satisfactory yells, cleared its own airway of amniotic fluid and mucus by crying and taking deep breaths, everyone sighed with relief. The period of silence and shushing was over. They turned up the operating room lights. The personnel began to talk loudly to each other. The baby was wrapped, introduced briefly to her mother and father. Then she was whisked away to the "safe" newborn nursery. I was so disappointed. The delivery was great, but the mother's opportunity to hold her baby and bond with her was not anyone's priority. We still had a long way to go to change medical practices.

Exploring Attachment

Our work on the early parent-infant relationship led into investigations into the development of attachment, which John Bowlby began exploring in the early 1960s. We identified four stages of attachment behavior between parent and infant prior to the stage that psychoanalyst Margaret Mahler called hatching at four and a half months. I later wrote about these stages with psychoanalyst Bertrand Cramer in *The Earliest Relationship*. The first stage is infants' achievement of control over outside stimuli and their own inner states and autonomic responses. Being able to attend to the sound and sight of another person requires this control. In the second stage, infants can prolong their attention and begin to interact with a caregiver. They learn to use cues from the adult to stay alert and adapt to the rhythm of a relationship. This stage may last from one to eight weeks. In the third stage, parents and infants can interact by building on the infant's ability to take in and respond to signals and to withdraw and recover. During this time, parents learn about their baby's skills and needs and his rhythm of attention-withdrawal-attention. They also learn about their own ability to draw the baby out. This stage takes place in the second or third month. In the fourth stage, babies begin to show their autonomy and recognize their control over their environment. A baby may stop during a feeding just to look around at something interesting. During this same time, at about four to five months, there is a leap in cognitive awareness. This roughly corresponds to the moment of infant "hatching."

These four stages of parent-infant attachment provided us as researchers with an opportunity to assess the quality of their relationship in the first four months. This research was instituted when I was a fellow at Jerome Bruner's lab at Harvard's Center for Cognitive Studies and became the base for identifying and understanding the behavior and rhythmic interaction that parents and babies also display in a typical office visit. Hence it could be used both diagnostically and as research data. The steps are incomplete or slowed down when parents are depressed or not attached or the infant is delayed or not responsive. Smiling, vocalizing, and motor behavior all fit into this frame. We made a film of the fourth stage of this behavior, with its violation, the so-called still-face situation designed by Ed Tronick to demonstrate the depth of attachment. In the film, the baby is shown responding enthusiastically to the mother. She then leaves the room and returns with a still face that does not change, whatever the baby does. The baby's intense efforts to woo her back and his joy when she responds again are striking. This film was so persuasive that it was shown at the House of Representatives and the US Senate in the mid-1980s to press for a parental leave bill. I describe these efforts in Chapter 7.

The NBAS Goes Abroad

Interest in the scale began to spread abroad. My first request was from Dr. Karl J. Scheppe at the University of Munich. He asked me to the university for a lecture. I spoke only a few words of German and was so nervous that I can hardly remember that visit. Thirty years later, in 2006, I revisited Munich with much more confidence when the Theodor Helbrügge Foundation, part of the University of Munich, honored me with the Arnold Gesell Prize.

My second invitation abroad came in 1974 from Dr. Peter Tizzard at Oxford. I was thrilled and anxious at being asked to give a lecture there. My dear friend, Aidan MacFarlane (a pediatrician who had been in Boston for training in child development), came from London to hear me. Jerome Bruner, my former boss at the Harvard Center for Cognitive Studies, had left Harvard and was then at Oxford, and he came and sat by my wife, Chrissy, in the front row.

Peter Tizzard was *the* professor of pediatrics and neonatology at Oxford and was very much feared and admired. I was terrified. I could hardly sleep. I certainly couldn't eat at the banquet they'd prepared for us. Everyone tried to reassure me, but by then I'd heard criticism of my work from Heinz Prechtl in Germany, from Peter Wolff at Harvard, and from various detractors of the NBAS in the Society for Research in Child Development (SRCD) and was already very defensive. I expected another beating. Reassured by Chrissy, Jerry, and Aidan, I steeled myself to march up with Tizzard, all decked out in robes and cap in the style of a major lecture at Oxford. A room full of eager faces. I had my film ready and showed it.

At the end of my talk, Professor Tizzard got up. "This is one of the most exciting breakthroughs in neonatology that I have ever witnessed." I began to beam proudly. Chrissy's face was skeptical. "BUT," he said, and the wind went out of me. "No one should use a repeated pinprick on a baby's foot. That's cruel." (This is an item in the NBAS to test a baby's response to pain.) I was too stunned to respond, to remind him that we are constantly pricking babies' feet for blood samples. However, he seemed genuinely impressed. Chrissy and Jerry were full of praise and reassured me that one never got just praise in England. It was always followed with a "BUT."

In 1973, the NBAS was published by Ronald Mac Keith of Mac Keith Press in London. Ronald was a brave godfather to the book, which we all doubted would ever pay for itself. However, it has gone through four editions and is translated widely.

The NBAS has since become known as the gold standard of infant assessment. It is used to assess newborns around the world. Kevin Nugent, a psychologist who joined me at Children's Hospital in 1978, has been leading teams of trainers. In addition to our work in the United States, there are nine training sites in Europe and others in Australia, Asia, and Latin America.

FOUR

Listening to Other Cultures

M y research with newborns led me to be curious about babies in other parts of the world. Everything suggested that they should be different—different genes, different nutrition, different experiences in utero, and different deliveries. Would babies in other cultures show differences in individual responses at birth? Would these in turn affect the way parents responded to them? Would different experiences over generations in the delivery and treatment of the new mother and her baby set practices that in turn lead to differences in behavior in the newborn and parent?

In the early 1960s, the documentary filmmaker Robert Gardner and his colleague Michael Rockefeller were going to New Guinea to record and to study war-making in remote parts of New Guinea. Bob came to tell me about it, and he said they were willing to take me along. I was thrilled, as I respected their work. After our discussion, and when we were beginning to plan, Bob said, "You'll have to stay over there with us for a year if you go." I suddenly realized, "But I can't go for a year, I have to make a living."

While I was deciding whether to go anyway, Margaret Mead came to my office. She was the most famous expert in our country on cross-cultural family life. I told her I was considering going to New Guinea (her old stomping ground) to see babies in these tribes. What did she think? "I don't think you'll get any chance to see a new baby over there unless you dress up in drag and paint your face," she said. Any culture protects its newborns, she explained. A man, especially a white one, would not be allowed to look at a vulnerable baby or enter a household of women. Then she looked me up and down and said, "Anyway, I wouldn't go if I were you. You look too succulent." So much for my dream of New Guinea. I had to refuse the offer.

Mayan Newborns in Southern Mexico

Not giving up on my dream to do cross-cultural assessments of newborns, however, in 1964 I sought out George Collier, an anthropologist and colleague of Evon Vogt, professor of anthropology at Harvard. George and his wife were bringing their own new baby on a field trip to study the Mayan babies of Zinacantán in Chiapas, southern Mexico, so he latched onto the chance of a pediatrician joining his research team. They had a project there, along with Stanford University. What an opportunity. Together with my wife and daughters, I figured I could go for a month each summer to see these babies in the highlands of Mexico. I could assess them as newborns, observe child-rearing practices, and see whether parents seemed to respond to their babies the way I would predict from their behavior.

It turned out, however, that none of their researchers had even seen Mayan newborns. No one was allowed to see a small baby less than three months of age who wasn't in on the delivery. Assessing their babies' development was difficult because mothers carried their babies in a serape on their backs. They covered their babies' faces and heads. After much wasted time in not being able to see babies or to play with small children, I grew frustrated. In Zinacantán the belief was strong that any stranger might have the evil eye and could damage the new baby without knowing it or meaning to be malevolent. Hence, no visits or assessments were allowed with either a pregnant woman or a new baby. Every time I tried to visit a pregnant woman, the thatched doors of her hut would be closed. If I tried to speak to a pregnant woman on the paths to Apas, the village (eight thousand feet above sea level) to which we were assigned, they hid their faces behind their hands and disappeared. My fourteen-year-old daughter, Kitty, helped. She learned Spanish and Tzotzil (the ancient Mayan tongue they still speak). She wore their clothes. She tied up her blonde hair in their headdress. In her company I managed to visit some families. My daughter could make eye contact with other young women, but I couldn't. No man would be allowed in another man's hut without a woman of his own family. Even toddlers and older children were afraid of me.

To make possible more observations, my anthropological colleague George Collier conceived of taking me to the home of one of his godchildren in Apas. He was accepted by them and their culture because he'd been down there for eight or ten years. Because I was with him, I was allowed in their household. The mother carried her baby, eight months old, on her back with his face and head covered. This mother turned carefully away from me to protect him. I carried a bright toy and held it within his sight. A little arm came out of the coverings to grab it. His mother slapped the hand, took away the toy to hand it back to me. Again, his little hand reached out to grab it.

Again, she took it away out of the blue. I said to her via a translator, "I'm a healer in my culture." She said, "We all know that—that is why we close our doors to you." Out of my mouth, unpremeditated came, "But if someone has the evil eye, I know how to cure it." The mother's eyes widened, her mouth dropped open. She pulled her baby out of the serape and handed him to me. I was amazed. He reached out, felt my mouth, and looked at me. After that she gave me permission to play with him. I tested him with my Bayley's toys (Bayley is a month-by-month infant test). He performed for me at an eight-month-old level for cognitive and motor development (object permanence, imitation as in peekaboo, recognizing a violation in the game of peekaboo, sitting alone and twisting around, creeping on his belly). Pulled to stand, he cooperated. I was delighted with him. Behind her shyness, so was his mother. By the time we left her household, there were at least four other mothers with babies waiting for me on the path. My "evil eye" ploy had worked! I've always wondered what would have happened if they'd held me to my brash statement. But their openness to me was miraculous afterward. I was able to play with their babies and to test them, and I was even invited to their households as long as Kitty came along. My acceptance had depended on my respecting their belief systems: (1) a stranger accepted only with a trusted person, (2) bringing a female family member to enter a household, and (3) the evil eye assertion. It was incredible how quickly my reputation as "safe and trustworthy" expanded. Other young parents were watching, listening, eager for safe communication with this strange white man. These belief systems, built up over the ages, were undoubtedly a way this strong tribe survived the centuries of invasion by the Spaniards. They probably helped protect vulnerable children from infection and women from molestation.

A Mayan Birth

Within the next few days, George Collier and I were invited to a delivery. It was at night, and the mother's whole family of sixteen was assembled. Everyone greeted me and my daughter with warmth and respect.

Zinacanteco cultural practices involving infant and child care are remarkably uniform. As in other cultures with extended families, knowledge is passed on directly by experienced older family members at the time of the birth and thereafter. No special rites and practices are carried out while a woman is pregnant, and no pharmacologic agents are given before or during delivery. Mary Anschuetz, in her field report "To Be Born in Zinacantan," describes the birth practice. The midwife, always present during childbirth, does not employ any particular obstetrical techniques but supports and encourages the mother in labor. Immediately after the birth, elaborate rituals are performed, with the newborn lying naked near the fire. Prayers and incantations by the midwife exhort the gods to bestow on the child all the manly or womanly attributes necessary for success in the Zinacanteco world. The child is then clothed. A long heavy skirt extending beyond the feet, which is worn throughout the first year by both sexes, is held in place by a wide belt or cinch wrapped firmly around the abdomen. Then the newborn is wrapped in additional layers of blankets to protect him from "losing parts of his soul." We observed that swaddling acts as a constant suppressant to reflexive motor activity. Infants' faces are covered in the presence of outsiders except during feedings, especially during the first three months.

At the delivery we attended, the young mother was having her first baby. Her husband was participating by pulling on a cinch around her waist, putting pressure on the fundus, or uppermost part of the uterus, to help her delivery. Her mother was kneeling before her and comforted her with each labor pain. A toothless old lady (the midwife) conducted a chorus of family and animals, with loud groans from all sixteen of the family, including the children and the animals, whenever she had a labor pain. Chickens and dogs that wandered in and out were also crowing and howling. The laboring mother was supported for each pain. She let out no protest herself. Her labor pains came every five to six minutes, and she seemed to be making progress.

The midwife's prayer for the soul of the baby seemed to reflect awareness of the very real precariousness of a new Zinacanteco life. When a boy is born, the tools and other work implements of a grown Zinacanteco man are placed in his hand. The midwife looks to the baby's future and values his gender and identity, evoking and reinforcing the cultural goal of the baby's adult male gender role. For girl babies, cooking, grinding, and weaving utensils and flowers are placed in her newborn grasp to enhance her future feminine role. The baby's value as a future member of society is emphasized.

After two hours, the elderly midwife became discouraged. She said that she must go home to her family, which was having a curing ceremony (the truth was she wasn't getting enough *pox*—grain alcohol). When she left, all the groans from the crowd ceased. Although there were plenty of elderly women present who could have and had conducted deliveries, no one stepped up to take over. The household became quietly depressed.

After a few more pains, the labor came to a stop. Everyone shook their bowed heads. A pall descended over the group. Even the chickens quieted down. I asked the family, "What's wrong? She was in hard labor before this." They said, "Her labor's stopped. The baby is stuck. It will probably die and she's going to die." I was horrified at their saying this in front of her. We would never make such an announcement in front of a patient in the United States, even if we knew it might be true. This energized me to want to help her. I said to her through my daughter's translation, "our women don't kneel for labor, as you are doing. When a woman's labor comes to a halt, we get her to walk around vigorously then she lays back and pushes on her uterus. That will usually start labor up again." The parents and her husband listened to me. They pressed her to comply. She walked around the hut two or three times, reluctantly, but without success. While she was being dutifully compliant, there was no labor.

After about two hours with mounting anxiety and sense of doom, the family sent out for another midwife. Another old woman walked in, took the larger bottle of *pox* that she was offered, and picked up her branch baton. She walked over to the pregnant woman and shook her vigorously. She said, "Now the baby is unstuck!" Sure enough, within a few minutes the labor pains began again. Everyone groaned along with them. Labor proceeded rapidly, and this young woman delivered a healthy baby in two hours. It seemed a miracle of psychosomatic medicine and of the role of belief in their culture. My suggestions had had no effect. It was another lesson in respecting different cultural beliefs and practices.

During the first month after delivery, the mother is confined, with the infant wrapped in her arms or laid supine beside her as she rests. Thereafter, the child is carried in a rebozo or serape on the mother or another woman's back when not feeding. Menda H. Blanco and Nancy Chodorow observed that siblings often care for infants, carrying them on their backs in imitation of the mother, rarely playing with them. Indeed, during the first year of life, I rarely saw them propped up to enable them to look around, nor did

I see them talked to or stimulated by eye-to-eye contact except by the mother.

A Quiet Infancy

Of course the Zinacanteco babies were breast-fed. In our US culture, a mother usually waits for her baby to signal that he is ready for feeding by crying and fussing. The mothers we saw in Mexico didn't wait for a cry. As soon as the baby became at all active, she'd pull the serape around to nurse the baby. If one breast didn't quiet his motor activity, she put him quietly to the other. We counted the number of breast feedings for these babies. They averaged eighty to ninety times per day. The goal for a feeding was apparently different in Zinacantán. It seemed to be aimed at keeping the baby quiet. In the United States, mothers generally wait until the baby's crying activity rouses him thoroughly. Then, she feeds him—reinforcing him for his own active participation. The goal of the Mayan mother was that of having a quiet, docile baby. She was protecting his low motor activity and high degree of sensitivity to stimuli from the first. These goals are completely different.

Babies were never put down on the dirt floors to crawl or to practice standing or walking. A common assumption in the United States is that in order for a toddler to learn to walk, he must test out each stage of motor learning. He must creep on his belly. He must pull up on furniture. He must practice day and night. Then he can put the different ingredients all together and start walking. In Zinacantán, without any of these experiences, babies walked at thirteen to fourteen months. Practicing and preparing for such a motor achievement was not a necessary part of their learning. They learned visually. The assumptions I'd been taught about motor development did not seem to fit this culture. We were impressed by the contrast to the way our babies learned. Playing with a baby to "teach" him a developmental step is not in the Zinacanteco repertoire. They expect a child to develop at his own pace. In addition, sex differences in socialization are started early. In the second year, boys and girls are already treated even more differently than they are in the United States. Boys were played with by older boys or with their fathers. Girls were assigned to women and girls in the family. If an older child played with a boy, he treated him differently than a girl. Everyone expected them to be different. Boys were expected to follow their fathers by four or five years of age and to work in the fields alongside them. They carried wood for their mothers. They never objected or rebelled. Even as toddlers, rebellion or temper tantrums were not part of their development. At most, a mild objection, but no negative behavior, was tolerated by adults.

A girl sat by her working mother all day. She was expected to help with tortilla making, with weaving, with household chores by four or five years. By eight or nine, a girl would watch over the younger children and wash the family clothes at the same time. A boy or a girl of eight would be trusted with the family fortune, the sheep herd, to watch all day.

And yet they were playful with each other, but quietly so. They told stories to each other. But only a father told stories to the whole family. Only a father could read. Mothers were expected to be workhorses. Fathers went to the village to trade and to sell goods, to make business. They dressed magnificently. Women wore the same *huipil* (shirt) day after day.

At birth, the babies were beautiful. They looked Asian (black hair, triangular faces, almond-shaped eyes, and slightly dark skin). In fact, when compared with babies I saw later in the Japanese Goto

Islands, they were so comparable that I couldn't help but feel that they were of an equivalent genotype.

These babies were remarkable for their quiet, graceful activity. Their movements were slow and measured, with very little jerky or startling activity. As a result of their motor activity having been restrained by swaddling, it seemed they were extremely sensitive to sensory stimuli. When I tested them with a red ball, they would alert right away and follow it, turning their heads. They turned immediately to a soft rattle and followed the sound back and forth with alert faces. A voice and face were even more interesting, and they'd follow my face back and forth for as long as thirty minutes without a break in attention. I was amazed, as I'd not been able to produce such prolonged attention in Caucasian newborns. Caucasian babies would alert, pay attention, and follow the stimulus. Then they would become excited and throw off a startle, which would interrupt their attention. If one waited and calmed them down, these Caucasian newborns could be brought back to pay attention to the stimulus. But never could I produce such a long attention span. The Mayan babies' ability to alert to a mother's or father's voice and face endeared them to their Mayan parents just as it does when I demonstrate it in the United States. The parents began to trust me more after I'd shared their babies' talents with them.

The babies remained highly sensitive to auditory and visual stimuli as they grew. Their mothers seemed to respond and to protect this high degree of sensitivity. The serape holding them provided a constantly soothing restraint as their mothers rocked back and forth all day grinding corn for tortillas. The auditory environment was quiet and protected their highly sensitive hearing. They were already gentle people, even as babies.

My question after this experience in Chiapas was this: Can their quiet, nonaggressive development as adults be attributed to their genetic background, or does their parents' response to the newborn's behavior cause them to develop the way they do? The development of children in Chiapas seems so economical—they do not need to have tantrums to establish their autonomy. They develop gently into their adult identity. They learn how to become effective, respected adults by imitation and visual learning. Visual learning is uppermost. Gender differences and conservation of energy are learned by three to four years. In our US culture, motor experimentation, more aggressive displays of rebellion (e.g., tantrums), and struggling to work toward individuality, though a more expensive model, are needed for becoming an effective adult.

This was a very traditional group of Mayan Indians who still practiced many of the ceremonies of the fifteenth century and still raised their children as they did in that era. They had successfully resisted the inroads of the Mexican government, Spanish culture, the Catholic Church, even Harvard and Stanford anthropologists. They resisted our influences by not accepting any changes without protecting themselves. For example, they used the Catholic Church as part of a ritual curing for an illness, but they surrounded it with three or four traditional curing ceremonies before and after the one at the church.

Behavior in Its Cultural Context

Clearly, the example of restricted motor movement in Zinacanteco newborns illustrates the adaptability of the baby to cultural practices. Even more important, it can reveal how a fit between the nature of the baby and infant care function to enhance survival in a particular niche of the physical environment. Note that swaddling is a successful adaptation to the cold. What if the Zinacanteco baby were very active and resisted swaddling? A newborn who kept kicking off his covers, as babies in the United States often do, would have a smaller chance of survival in the cold climate of highland Chiapas in a house that goes totally unheated during the night.

While overall scores in our assessments in Zinacantán generally lagged about one month behind norms established in the United States, the lag was consistently greater for motor skills than for cognitive skills. Yet the inborn program for motor development drives the baby on in spite of little practice and what we think of as direct reinforcement from the environment. The close tactile and kinesthetic stimulation from being carried all day on the mother's back serves as the necessary sensory input or fuel for the developmental program to proceed. Female observers have noted that babies are played with in a one-to-one or face-to-face situation when no males were present. Our observations as male observers may be influenced by these gender-linked customs. In any event, these infants were understimulated from the point of view of our culture, but not for their needs. Jerome Kagan's observations in Guatemala where he thought (as we did) that babies were less stimulated, bears out our own observations. The fact that those babies, as ours, developed in a universal maturational sequence without marked delay in motor or cognitive development bears out both the importance of (1) the inborn maturational program and (2) alternative ways of fueling that development. Other modalities than face-to-face or motor stimulation can fuel successful development in infancy.

Robert LeVine notes that survival of the infant is an overriding cultural value in societies in which there is a high infant mortality rate. In such societies (of which Zinacantán is one) survival overrides goals of optimizing development. Surviving the cold is more important than speeding up motor development. Hence, what we might consider a deficit from our point of view becomes an advantage in the ecological niche occupied by another society.

Indeed, the Zinacantecos do not seem interested in "optimizing" motor development. Based on an intensive study of ten Zinacanteco families, Francesco Cancian reports that "for babies, as for older children, there is little pressure from adults to master basic skills, and little pride on the part of parents over the speed with which their children learn to walk or talk." Given this attitude, it is interesting that Zinacanteco babies lagged only one month behind American norms in developmental testing (especially considering how foreign the tests were to them: e.g., Zinacanteco infants are never placed in the prone position required for certain motor items).

For the Zinacantecos we studied, a key concept was *baz'I*, the true way, synonymous with the Zinacanteco way. In order to maintain the "true way" in the face of influences from modernization and the surrounding Latino community, it must be transmitted to the next generation in every area of life—work roles, familial roles, religious roles. Also, as we came to realize through our developmental research, the culture not only transmits the *content* of socialization, it transmits *processes* of learning and teaching that maximize cultural continuity and minimize deviation. The first such process to appear in infancy is imitation of a model.

The innate foundation of skill in imitating a model lies in the Zinacanteco newborn's unusual attentiveness and sensitivity to visual and auditory stimuli: the first step in imitating a model is to observe and comprehend it. Pediatrician John Robey, George Collier, and I saw their excellent ability to imitate in the developmental testing we did from one to nine months of age. Repeatedly,

infants watched us carefully as we demonstrated the use of test objects, and then they imitated each movement we had made to
score a success on the test. Then they would drop the object without any of the exploration or experimental play we would have
seen in US babies.

While novelty, exploration, and experimentation are highly valued in our culture, they constitute a danger to a culture that wants
to transmit a replication of itself to the next generation. A possible
outcome of exploration, experimentation, and attraction to novelty is innovation and change. Hence, these are not reinforced by
parents in Chiapas as babies play with objects.

Nutrition and Infant Development in Guatemala

After my experience in Zinacantán with the Mayan descendants, I
published several papers on babies and early development there.
Evon Vogt's group from Harvard was pleased, as little had been
known about Mayan early childhood. As a result, our work became
known to anthropologists and infant researchers. In 1971, I got a
call from Robert Klein, who led a study of the effects of malnutrition
on babies' development in the eastern slopes of Guatemala. He had
a grant from INCAP (Instituto de Nutrición de Centro América y
Panamá) and WHO to study four villages—two of which would be
offered nutritional supplements, two of which would be used as controls. It had been determined that pregnant women there were ex-
isting on 1200 calories a day, whereas a diet for pregnant women in
the United States was thought to be 2200 calories. Studies had
shown that adequate nutrition during pregnancy is necessary for a
normal brain at birth. I was given the chance to evaluate the newborns from these two groups of four villages.

When we arrived in this eastern part of Guatemala, we were stunned at the poverty. There were few tilled fields. Streets were dusty and empty; houses were made of rotting wood. The children were emaciated and almost lifeless. The toddlers and small children had the reddish hair of kwashiorkor (a severe nutritional deficiency disease seen in Africa and other desperately undernourished parts of the world). After weaning from breast milk, the toddlers developed swollen bellies, matchstick limbs, and lifeless faces. In this condition, many of them died from minor infections. They had few or no antibodies to fight disease. An estimated 40–50 percent of children in each family were liable to die in infancy and early childhood. The women had no knowledge of pregnancy prevention or of how to space children. They were likely to deliver again early in the second year, although they were still breast-feeding the first baby. Once they realized they were pregnant, they either weaned the first child or began to give him fewer feedings. As a result, the toddler sensed his new deprived role and his depression added another insult to his extremely marginal nutritional state. By the time he was fully weaned at eighteen months to make way for the second baby, he was already likely to have kwashiorkor and be open to disease.

In these villages, one saw few children playing—no running around or laughter or calling to each other. Even the dogs were skinny and listless, cowering if we went close to them. We began to realize that dogs in a village reflected the nutritional status as clearly as the children did. As the children grew, they were always several inches below the expected height of US children. Average adult height was about five feet to five feet two. No adult was likely to be even as tall as five feet, four inches. Malnutrition was stunting their growth, their brain development, their immunity, and any ability to drive themselves to find a job or any future expectation that they might be successful in life. Here, a grown man would work at most a few hours a day. A woman would cook a simple meal once a day, but her chores were limited as she went from one demanding pregnancy to the next. The general atmosphere in these villages was that of depression and hopelessness.

The research program called for giving a nutritional supplement to the pregnant women in two of the villages. The supplement was called Incaparina and contained six hundred calories, which were supposed to bring up the pregnant women's intake closer to two thousand calories a day. All pregnant women were herded in to partake of this rather foul-tasting liquid. I noted that instead of dutifully accepting it as it was doled out to them, the women would bring out a vessel from under their skirts. They'd pour the liquid into the vessel to take it home. It took us some time to realize what was happening. Because they were told the liquid was nutritious, the women wanted to share it with the rest of their families. In other words, the supplement was not reaching the mother or fetus. Her role was to feed her family, not herself. The education we offered about how important this supplement was had taken hold, but it was not doing the job we'd hoped of nourishing the fetus and its developing brain.

As a result, at birth, the newborns like those in other villages were small for their delivery dates. They weighed two to three kilograms (4–6.5 pounds) and were slightly long and lean. They looked worried, even at birth. When we assessed them on my neonatal scale (NBAS), they scored poorly on nearly all the items. They were difficult to rouse; they moved sluggishly from one state to another. Their extremities were weak and somewhat limp because their muscle tone was poor. As they were handled, they cried weakly and responded with dull, wide eyes. All in all, not very rewarding for their already overloaded, poor parents.

When we asked new mothers how often they breast-fed these infants, they responded, "Whenever they want." When we observed in their homes, we found that this amounted to three to four times in a twenty-four-hour day at a time when six to eight feedings are necessary for normal development. In other words, malnutrition during pregnancy resulted in undemanding babies whose mothers therefore responded to them with fewer feedings. Whatever toll malnutrition had taken on their brain development in utero was reinforced with this unresponsiveness as newborns, leading to poor nutrition. The vicious cycle of poverty was set up again: hopelessness, poor brain development, and listlessness from one generation to another.

Mealtime in these households was interesting in that the relatively more vigorous, aggressive children got the most food from the common feeding vessels—contributing to their better development. The well-fed children became the leaders and were more intelligent. The less well fed became more and more passive, falling behind. Leadership was connected with nutrition.

A follow-up of all the children at ages six and seven demonstrated that their IQ performances averaged 85 and varied from 75 to 90. In other words, at school age, their IQs were 10–15 points below the expected average for children around the world. School success was already less likely for these children. In addition, they stayed smaller than they might have been, an inch or two already, and were more prone to infection. Every organ had likely been affected by deprivation during pregnancy and the early months.

We learned from our mistaken design of offering supplement to a mother in pregnancy. Maternal concern for the children she already had superseded the mother's own need for calories. Roberto Chavez in Mexico in association with Joaquin Cravioto conducted a parallel experiment that was successful. They were more innovative and had anticipated the failure we met in offering supplements. They explained to pregnant women that if they wanted a smart baby in the future, they would have to drink the supplement themselves. Their babies turned out to be responsive and had IQs (95–100) closer to the world average. As children, they were more energetic and more successful in first grade. That study along with ours seemed to confirm that supplemental nutrition for pregnant women who are otherwise poorly fed helped the physical and cognitive well-being of their newborns. Given such extra nutrition in utero, babies became more demanding, leading to mothers feeding them six to eight times a day. Good nutrition leads to more alert, responsive, rewarding babies and more responsive mothers too. The vicious cycle of undernutrition can be broken. Alert, demanding babies grow into children more successful in school and who become better prepared to take leadership roles in their communities. As a result of this study, those of us participants speculated whether nutritional failure might have been one of the variables in the downfall of the Mayan culture.

Playing with Kenyan Newborns

In 1975, Ed Tronick and I joined anthropologist Robert LeVine in a study of child development in Kisii, Kenya. The Gusii of Kisii live between the Masai and Lake Victoria in western Kenya. They are a farming culture. Land is their most valuable commodity. At the time we were there, polygamy was legal. Land was becoming fragmented into less and less useful plots. Each woman tilled her own but could barely feed her children. The birthrate was among the highest in the world (at that time, eleven per woman). Despite a poor infant survival rate, supporting a family on the meager land was nevertheless a major problem.

Bob LeVine's book *Child Care and Culture: Lessons from Africa* summarizes our experience there. We had been planning for a year or more before we went. We had representatives from medicine, psychology, and anthropology in our group. That gave us a wonderful chance to share ideas and observations. Bob had done anthropological studies in West Africa; Sarah, his wife, had done a women's study; and Herbert and Gloria Liederman (psychiatrist and psychologist) had studied California families and done cross-cultural work. Charles Super, a psychologist, and Sarah Harkness, an educator and anthropologist, were to join us from Harvard School of Education. They and the Liedermans would split off to study a more northern tribe in Kenya.

I was training pediatricians at Harvard, and two of my trainees, Constance Keefer, MD, and Suzanne Dixon, MD, were eager to go and conduct a pediatric clinic in Kisii in order to give medical care to the community. We wanted to evaluate the babies at birth, follow them monthly with physical exams, and study the child-rearing practices by sitting in their huts with them to observe day after day. We wanted to be able to design appropriate studies of early development, of attachment, and of the effects of nature and of nurture.

Playing with the Kenyan newborns was fun! They used their bodies to cling to you right from the first. Pulled to sit by their arms, newborns would come up to stand, maintain themselves in standing, look around the room as if saying, "There's my new world. I want to conquer it!" If you played with them, they'd almost laugh, so delighted were they with exciting motor responses. Rocking them up and down alerted them. Even in a standing position, a newborn would alert, follow my face, and turn to my voice. As long as one played with them, they remained excited and alert.

This ability to be excited by motor activity persisted right through the first year. The babies would giggle, wanting to imitate and be imitated. (Peekaboo was also a favorite game in the last half of the first year.)

Their mothers expected their babies to be responsive. They would pick them up, plant them on their hips, and wrap a dashiki around themselves and the baby. They'd leave the neck and head free. The infants responded by adjusting to an upright position on their mothers' bodies, maintaining their heads from the first. They perked up when their mothers played with them. They were different babies from the ones we'd played with in Guatemala.

Suzanne's husband, Michael Hennessy, MD, an orthopedic surgeon, was eager to study the precocity in their early motor development—how they learned to sit, and then to walk. Was it different from US babies, who were more delayed, took more practicing, and so on? What did their earliest experience with being handled and expected to sit and stand early have to do with this precocity? To study this, he attached luminous patches onto each joint in order to film their motion in the dark. He found that they did little practicing to be ready. They just seemed to stand up and start walking. No practicing like our babies did. As they began, they were clumsier and less agile at protecting themselves from falling. They walked stiffly with a wider base, straight legs, and were awkward for a while. But even by about nine months, they could stand and walk for long periods without tiring. Motivation for motor activity was high, and they seemed proud of their ability to master their arms and legs. Babies of this age in the United States have more delicate, agile fingers and toes. They have more time to develop fine motor skills since they have less interference at this age from large motor activity. Although there was a range of individual differences, depending on temperament, as there is in the United States, the average timing of each motor milestone was significantly earlier for Kenyan babies. No one expected them to sit alone or to crawl, because they were carried all day long. But when they were "ready," they walked. They didn't protest as our babies do for autonomy, but parents seemed proud of their readiness for walking and were eager to encourage it. The parents probably got certain signals when the child was ready.

In Kisii, Kenya, we saw how a baby's motor interaction was already mixed with social interaction. At home, everyone played with them. As a result, motor development continued to be unexpectedly advanced. They were never walked or stood per se but it happened all the time in play. I noticed a seated grandmother who was playing with her baby granddaughter. I said, "She seems to be trying to walk." "Oh yes, she's five months old, and she can walk." "Five months! I can't believe it!" She motioned for me to sit about six feet away. She got the baby to use her walk reflex then let her go toward me. This five-month-old baby maintained her body posture and tottered over about six steps into my arms. I could hardly believe it. Through a translator, I questioned the grandmother, "How many months since she came?" "Five." It was surely hard to believe. But most babies were walking by seven or eight months. I never saw them put down to crawl. They got themselves upright and just started walking.

Because they live on dirt floors and have a center fire burning all the time, children are not encouraged to crawl. They are rarely put down on the ground. The whole family's attention to motor achievements is reinforcing and responsive to the motor excitement present in the newborns from the first. They encourage him, clap for him, and limit his explorations so he cannot hurt himself. Young children, as early as four and five years, are learning how to parent a baby. An older child, eight or ten, can take over. At twelve to fourteen, the sexes separate, and boys are no longer babysitters. Girls often become wives by fourteen or fifteen, so they must be ready. Because they all eat out of the same pot, we watched to see how a two- or three-year-old was fed. He was likely to be clumsy, and the older children made a bit of a special place for him, encouraging him, often even feeding him with their fingers. No eating problems that we could see. Food was such a form of communication in these families. They were too close to the edge of famine, and food had a very special meaning to them.

All of the children slept together. The baby slept between the parents until the mother was several months pregnant with the next baby. Then, she'd put him out of her bed, stop breast-feeding him, and expect him to learn to care for himself. His siblings then felt responsible for him. He usually slept in a common bed with them—they comforted him.

When I came back from these experiences in Kenya, I wanted to see if they related to those of parents in my practice. I wondered why they didn't let their children run around more. But in the United States, when being read to or taught in any way, children are expected to be sitting down. Even though many young children do better when "taught on their feet," many preschools have not picked this up. Some American parents worry that a child who is precocious motorically wouldn't be as intellectually competent. There is no substance to such concerns. Nor does motor precocity lead to hyperactivity. Children who are motoric in temperament learn best on their feet. I realized that we needed to change our early educational systems to adapt to such differences in children.

Infancy and Early Attachment in Japan

In 1983, I was invited by the Japanese government and my friend Noburu Kobayashi to come to Japan. Noburu (or Kobey, as we called him) and I had met at various international conferences. A pediatrician, he held a high position in the government, involved in infant health. When he learned about my scale, he sent one of his students to be trained. Noburu wanted him to train Japanese doctors to use the NBAS all over Japan. Noburu had a great friend and advocate, Mr. Masaru Ibuka, the former CEO of Sony. He was powerful and very interested in fostering Japanese awareness of the importance of infancy and of early attachment of parents to their infants. He saw that Japan was about to change, with more and more women in the workforce, and he wanted to be sure to protect the mother-child relationship.

An unusual event in Japan had taken place: it was reported that over a period of two years, several eight- and nine-year-old boys had killed their mothers. These tragedies were blamed on the intense desire for upward mobility among Japanese parents. They pushed, pushed, pushed their children to get into the right child-care center, the right preschool, the correct grade school, and the right secondary school. When the child didn't make it, some became so upset that they killed the only person they could blame: their mothers. This was absolutely frightening to the Japanese government, as well it should have been. Mr. Ibuka and Dr. Kobayashi made plans to get an unusual team of experts together to travel all over Japan, talking about early attachment and its importance. Jane Goodall, who worked at the Gombe Reserve in Africa for chimpanzees and may well know more about chimpanzee nurturing than anyone in the world, was invited. A famous Australian child psychiatrist, Paul Campbell; a French educator; and Chrissy and I were to go.

When we arrived in Japan, we were housed in a fabulous old inn. The rooms were traditional Japanese: mats on the floor on which we slept; paper walls, which we rolled back to go from one room to another; bathrooms with squatting toilets. So many things to learn in a new culture! The paper walls were magnificent, with very subtle designs, but one could hear everything from one room to another. We got to know each other better than we had expected.

The four of us "experts" went from city to city in Japan: Tokyo, Kyoto, Osaka, Nagasaki. Jane talked about her chimp babies in just the way I talked about our human babies. She showed how she held them gently out in front of her, to talk to them face to face. She had superb films of chimp mothers and even fathers nurturing their babies in the wild. What a delight it was to compare notes with her. As we went around to each city, hundreds of parents gathered for each presentation. None of us could speak Japanese, but that didn't seem to dampen the enthusiasm. We were told that we were making an impact on Japanese parents. Hard to believe.

In Osaka, a prominent private researcher took Chrissy and me out to his reserve so we could observe nonhuman parent-infant interaction "in the wild." In Nagasaki, an orthopedic surgeon, Dr. Tomitaro Akiyama, introduced himself. He had translated the NBAS into Japanese and taught people to use it. In Japan, he explained, orthopedists are responsible for early intervention with children with special needs. He was interested in starting early intervention with these children from birth onward. At his hospital, they did very well in making up for motor delays, but he said that the children didn't "make the progress he'd like in cognitive and emotional development because their parents won't stay involved." "Especially on the Goto Islands off the coast," he said, "we can't get parents interested enough to bring their children to us for early intervention." He asked for our help.

Of course, I was intrigued and challenged. I assured him that I was ready to help, but, in order to be of any real use, I'd have to understand the culture much better than I did. "Would you be interested in coming to help us study these babies?" Of course I would, but I told him that we'd have to plan ahead for it, because I had a heavy teaching load at Harvard. He assured me that it would be possible and asked me to come the following year to study the babies and the culture on the Goto Islands. I could live there for a month at a time.

The Goto Islands are part of a chain in the Pacific from Okinawa to Korea. There are 140 islands in all, 5 main ones. (*Goto* means "five" in Japanese.) They were the last stops for sailing ships before leaving for China. They were undeveloped, still traditional fishing islands. Their whole economy is fishing. The men fish; the women mend nets and clean fish.

My son, Tom, and I went. We lived on the main island, Fukue, for a month. We enlisted thirty newborns for our study. At birth, the newborns were sturdy, beautiful, quiet babies who paid attention for prolonged periods. Their movements were liquid and gentle, and their fingers and toes were freely involved in their ballet-like movements. Like the Mayan babies, they were born and raised in the context of low-keyed motor activity, and so a newborn would pay attention to a soft rattle, a red ball, or your face for as long as thirty minutes without a break. I had been able to produce at most three to five minutes of tracking and listening in US newborns. This difference in the ability to pay prolonged attention was amazing to me, representing differences in genetic endowment and early environment. I decided to see how basic this prolonged attention would be if the environment were different. In the Goto Islands, women were quiet, slow moving, and never exposed to loud noises or activity. So I also observed mothers and infants in Tokyo. There, women were dashing around amid loud noises, traffic, and the like. Their newborns still had long attention spans, but not thirty minutes. They managed about eighteen minutes without a break. Later, a study of Asian babies in San Francisco showed that a newborn's attention span there was down to twelve minutes. We felt this was a great example of the effects of experience before birth in shaping the behavior of the newborn.

Mothers in the Gotos walk slowly and live a quiet life. They talk to each other in low-pitched voices. Tension is not high in the Goto Islands, as far as we could observe. The fetus's experience during pregnancy is a gentle, calm, well-fed one. In Tokyo, mothers are under much more stress. They walk differently; they rush to cross an intersection, looking up and down then hurrying across the street. All day, their movements and lives are more punctuated with jerky, tense movements, and stressful, noisy events. These provide the fetus with a different experience than that in the Gotos. In San Francisco, the effects of a stressfully active life are even greater. Nature and nurture already work together to create differences at birth. Add these to the effects of very different lives ahead. It isn't hard to visualize the different kind of adults this will produce.

The Goto mothers (who had been mending nets and cleaning fish until they delivered) stayed in the hospital for seven days. Then they were sent to their mothers' homes. There, they were expected to regress completely. Wrapped in a futon, each with her baby next to her, they were treated as babies themselves for one month. Their only job was to feed their babies. When they needed to go to the toilet, someone helped them. They were fed by chopsticks "like a baby." Spoken to in baby talk, they responded in baby talk. Chisato Kawasaki, a pediatrician who was with us, documented the fact that there were no postpartum depressions after this early treatment. In Japan, a new mother could regress to her own babyhood for one month.

The thirty newborns we evaluated on the Goto Islands were half from fishing families, half white collar. We scored them by their performance on the NBAS, especially for their responsiveness to faces and voices and to nonhuman stimuli, for their motor fluidity and competence, and for their ability to soothe themselves when they were upset. We planned to see whether these scores predicted how well the babies would do on cognitive tasks later on. We returned every two years to evaluate them. At first we used the Bayley exam, later the Stanford-Binet. Each year, these exciting babies maintained high scores. The children all progressed equally through the third year. Then, half of them continued to make optimal progress on the test scores, but the other half began to level off and even to lose levels of IQ functioning by the age of five. Those babies who lost IQ, however, were well equipped to respond, and, with pressure, extra time, and assurance, they could achieve the higher levels of their peers. It became apparent that it was not the ability to achieve optimal scores but the motivation and the excitement of being tested that were significantly different. The white-collar parents who wanted their children to succeed in the corporate world of Japan were pushing them—four-year-olds in preschool, then school. The fishing parents were not pushing their children to perform cognitively. They expected them to stay on the island and fish. The potential of the child in the cognitive area was not their measure of success.

When we returned several years later, the fisherman's children were in school, but relaxed, content with joining their parents in their traditional work. Children pressed by their parents were likely to be tense, often with problem behavior. Many of them had gone to the mainland to be prepared for high-powered careers and thus were already out of touch with their families.

Dr. Akiyama was very grateful for the ideas we could give him about how to work with new parents. We agreed that the time to capture them for early intervention if their baby was likely to have special needs was soon after birth. Then, sharing with parents the work necessary for early intervention would be a way to approach these isolated people. It meant that we had to train a pediatrician or neurologist (or orthopedist) from Fukuoka to evaluate all newborns for any neurological impairment or any question about development that showed up on my newborn assessment. Akiyama was eager to institute this, and the Nagasaki University School of Medicine became a very active site for training physicians from the islands as well as from all over Japan. They are still an active NBAS site and have published many papers on its use for diagnosis and prediction.

Dr. Akiyama arranged for Kevin Nugent to join me on our visits every two years. We helped his Nagasaki staff train eight to ten physicians each time. Meanwhile, we'd go to the Gotos each visit and follow up on our original babies. We grew devoted to all the Nagasaki team: Shohei Ogi, Chisato Kawasaki, and Tomitaro Akiyama.

China: Observing the One-Child Family

In 1983, UNICEF called me to represent SRCD as a member of a team to go to Beijing to study the effects of the one-child family policy that the Chinese government was instituting. This was in an effort to control the enormous population explosion. In Beijing, millions of émigrés from the countryside poured into the already crowded city. No one had cars; bicycles filled streets and sidewalks. There was the same transportation gridlock with bicycles on the main streets in Beijing that you witness with automobiles in a city like Los Angeles. The growing population threatened to overwhelm China's resources.

In a culture that had been intergenerational, needing the younger generation to care for the elderly, each couple in a marriage now needed to take care of two sets of grandparents. Most Chinese wives work. The national need was too great not to include women as well as men in the workforce. But then, how to care for the one child? Grandparents were working too. Child-care centers were rapidly being organized. Wages were low; training of child-care workers had not been instituted in China. Families had relied on the extended generations.

My SRCD colleagues and I met almost daily to complete our study. We compared three- and four-year-olds who were being raised in one-child families with children from two-child families (there were still plenty of these available). We compared them on (1) how narcissistic they were, (2) whether they ever shared toys or think about other children, and (3) whether other three- and four-year-olds liked them. In this controlled study, the child from one-child families scored more poorly on each item. Everyone said, "Of course. They are spoiled by six adults (two parents and four grandparents) who submit to every whim. This child feels he's the center of the universe." (Though this was the concern at that time, subsequent research has shown that only children are not necessarily so spoiled. They still are raised to respect their elders and be oriented to the needs of others.) As we presented these findings to a group of psychologists and administrators, I was seated next to a Mrs. Lee, whose husband was a top official in the government. Mrs. Lee turned to me, to say, "This will never work for Communism, will it?" I had to agree. The small group began to examine the consequences of these findings and what they might do about them. The Chinese authorities suggested keeping grandparents of one-child families away from the child. Then, they wouldn't be so spoiled. Nodding heads. I couldn't help but pipe up: "But in a country where tradition and intergenerational values are so critical, what message will you be giving?" Again, they all nodded.

Another suggestion was to take the babies away from their "spoiling" environments when they are too young to have gotten spoiled. Put them in day care by four months. I piped up again: "You are already asking parents to give up desired future babies. You are asking them to invest themselves in this one very precious baby. What do you think that it will mean to parents to have to give up that one child to child care as early as that?" The marvelous thing about China then was that they were seeking solutions, but they hadn't necessarily made up their minds, at least about what only one child will mean to parents. The authorities in our group listened. Their solution took each objection into account. Not only did they try to provide better child care for working women, they worked to free up grandparents from their jobs so that they could care for their grandchildren. Maybe it wouldn't work for all families, but the grandparents would have the choice.

In 1984, I was sent to follow up on the effects of this change and to teach for a month. First, we went to Shanghai. The head of pediatrics was a short, winning man named Guo Di, who dominated the pediatric department at the General Hospital in Shanghai. He probed me for my interests, my research, my writing. Later, he had *Infants and Mothers* translated into Chinese. They called it the

"Golden Book" for parents to learn about child development and published it with a gold cover. Though it was not clear what an American book on child rearing would mean to Chinese parents, the book was well received and will appear in a new edition in 2013.

While we were in Shanghai, Guo Di and I became fast friends. He taught me about the Chinese Communist culture—pros and cons. I taught him about child development. He began to incorporate these ideas into his training of pediatricians and teaching. The Shanghai Hospital had the second-largest children's service in the country, so his influence was powerful.

Before we left, the hospital gave us a candlelit, six-course dinner in the basement of the hospital. We all dressed up and sang songs together. A resident played the lute and sang haunting songs about China's history. Others sang the marching songs of Mao Zedong. We talked openly about the past, what was given up, and the promise of the future. Everyone saw China as having a brilliant future. No one seemed to resent the edict of a one-child family.

We went on to Beijing where, as representatives of SRCD, we taught about babies in the Capital Hospital as well. Ji Xiao Cheng was a professor of pediatrics at the hospital. A tall, handsome, affable man, obviously wellborn, he had studied in San Diego with Dr. Lou Gluck, a famous neonatologist in the United States. He learned the NBAS and taught one of his students, Bao Xiu-lan, how to administer and to teach it. The two of them published several papers in US journals and many in the Chinese pediatric journals based on the use of my scale. They saw to it that I had a chance to play with many Chinese newborns. There, I experienced the same neonatal behavioral differences that I had experienced in Japan: quiet, gentle, very competent motor movements; less upset states, crying easy to console;

highly responsive to auditory and visual stimuli, many of them even hypersensitive in these areas; long periods of attention, of turning their heads easily to follow an object or one's face.

On a later trip, intrigued by these quiet, gentle, sensitive babies, I asked to spend daylight hours watching in homes as parents (and grandparents) handled and reared them. The babies made it easy to relate to the adults. I went to several tiny apartments to observe. I would sit for six to eight hours taking notes on everything that happened.

I remember one apartment that seemed rather typical except that the mother was a movie star. She and her husband lived in a two-room apartment with a tiny bath and kitchen between the two rooms. Each room was about ten by ten feet and had a bed in it. The grandparents lived in one room, the young parents in the other. They had a nine-month-old boy who had just begun to crawl. He was dressed in a little jacket that buttoned at the neck and pants that were split up the back to facilitate toileting, as is the tradition in China. Every few hours or so, he was seated upon a little pot, in his mother's lap, until he produced. Sometimes it was an hour of sitting and waiting. No play, no reading, just concentrating on his "job." When he finally produced urine or feces, he was rewarded by being allowed his freedom to move about. That meant he was placed on his parents' double bed. He could creep and crawl on it. As he got too close to the edge of the bed, his parents would pull him back to the center. Freedom to move meant the freedom to explore a plain environment like the parents' bed. No one ever put him on the floor or encouraged him to stand or to move freely. It was a very controlled environment.

As I commented on his desire to move around and his ability to creep and even to crawl (up on his hands and knees), his young mother beamed. She seemed so pleased at my approval of his motor development that she admitted: "We are trying to raise him like a boy in America, lots of freedom and independence. Do you think there is anything that you do that we should be doing to assure that?" How could I answer her? There was no correlation between the environment in which he was being raised and the one we provided in our country. There was already a combination of nature and nurture that was bound to shape him as a person with different values from ours.

Babies in the United States are more vigorously motoric at birth. They love to be played with in active ways. They develop a negativism by nine months that wouldn't have made it as easy for this mother to restrict her baby had she had an American baby. But because she had an Asian baby and her customs led her to refuse the kind of exploration and hence the number of choices, her baby was more docile and didn't fall apart at an age when that might have been expected in the United States. His genes and his environment were playing together to produce a quietly compliant toddler.

In one home, I observed a two-year-old climbing on a sofa. As he clambered to the top, teetering, and might have been in danger, his mother said from across the room, "Get down." And he did! She had control of this toddler and clearly understood him. I wondered whether this earlier experience of restricted motor behavior made it likely that a child develops with limited expectations and, marvelously, the ability to find satisfaction in other skills. The children I observed were extremely good with fine motor skills. They could almost draw a figure and could write their name by the age of two. These children demonstrated a kind of passive compliance and necessary self-control over their rebellious feelings. The example of a mother's control over her toddler on the bed was an example. This suppression of rebellious feelings and the quiet passivity on the surface made the movie-star mother's desire for an American-style freedom unlikely to be fulfilled. For the Chinese, a child who cares mainly about himself and isn't interested in pleasing is thought of as "spoiled."

On that trip, I stood on the corner in Beijing, counting the number of blue and the number of pink decorated baby strollers. About the same number. But it couldn't last. Under the one-child policy, boys were so much more highly valued that girls were given up for adoption in other countries. Also, a technique for early intrauterine diagnosis of the sex of the babies had been developed, making abortion of female babies possible. Families with one child were likely to be families with little boys.

On another occasion, I went to a first-grade class in Beijing with Harold Stevenson, a professor of education from the University of Michigan. The teachers taught by acting out the lessons they wanted the children to learn. They expected these Chinese six-year-olds to learn visually, by modeling. The teachers watched the children's eyes for evidence that they had learned each bit of material. Their eyes would brighten and the teacher knew the children had understood it. After forty-five minutes of such passive learning, the teacher and the students were exhausted. The children were sent outside to play actively. The teacher used the fifteen-minute break from each hour to recover herself. After fifteen minutes of active and noisy play, the children came back together in the classroom for quiet, visual learning. Both teacher and child were ready for this regeneration at the end of each hour of schoolwork. This rhythm certainly reinforced the kind of steady development one observed in Chinese children as they grew.

Tradition and Trust: Among the Navajos

In 1983, I was asked to Gallup and Shiprock in New Mexico to work with newborns among Navajo in Arizona. One of my old trainees at Children's, Jeremy Mann, was in charge of the Navajo hospital at Tuba City. In addition, I knew the head of social work at Chinle, one of the main villages. I ended up visiting Chinle, Shiprock, and Tuba City for nearly a week, demonstrating newborn behavior to the staff at each hospital. I met the head nurse, Ursula Wilson, a Navajo who told me about Navajo traditions. We became good friends, and she appreciated various suggestions I made as we toured the hospital. She asked me whether I'd like to attend a special ceremony with peyote as the "cure" for the whole community. It was to be attended by a healer, and few who were not Navajo had ever been asked before. About ten of us sat around in a circle. Each of us held chicken bones and feathers, which were specially blessed by the curer. A pipe of peyote was passed around as the Navajos chanted blessings with each other. The pipe was passed round and round, obviously very sacred to them. Each time, I acted as if I puffed on it. Even being engulfed in its smoke made my head dizzy. I was told that having been included in such a ceremony, I was an "adopted Navajo." I was respectfully seeping up everything that I could.

Ursula was obviously a powerful person. She later became head of nurses in the Navajo community. As we went from one hospital to another, being with her gave me status. The new hospital at Window Rock was a great asset, but it wasn't as strong in native motifs as Ursula and I wanted. They finally developed one room for sand painting in which the patients could come and do a painting to record their dreams of conquering illness. Their vision of recovery turned out to be a breakthrough. Children vied with each other to do a sand painting. Afterward, it was reported that their "get well" time was significantly reduced. They left with more joy and less anxiety. "Patient satisfaction" rates increased markedly. Incorporating part of the Navajo tradition turned out to be an effective way of dealing with feelings of hopelessness and helplessness in an otherwise Anglo-appearing hospital.

In Tuba City, I was invited to demonstrate an assessment on a Navajo newborn to the staff of Anglo physicians and Navajo nurses. I asked to have the mother participate, believing that this could increase the chances of the mother communicating with the staff. "Navajos never speak." "They never ask a question." "I don't feel I have any relationships with them," I was told by the Anglo physicians. I hoped the newborn could break down that barrier between them.

We took the newborn from the nursery to his mother's bedside. Although I wasn't sure how much English she spoke, I asked for her permission to show what her baby could do. I had been warned that I should *not* look at her baby in the face, because a new mother would be frightened that I could damage her baby. I was aware of the cultural taboos and intended to respect them, so I asked her at each stage whether it was permitted for me to try out each of my assessment behaviors on her baby. As I expected, she was very quietly passive and guarded. I knew she was too frightened to say "no." I took each step very slowly and quietly, watching her out of the corner of my eye. Everyone in the hospital gathered to watch the baby perform his visual and auditory miracles.

The baby boy was just wonderful, gentle, alert and responsive. As I played with him, I got more and more excited. So did he. So did his mother. She was sitting up in her bed, watching and admiring everything he did. As he turned to watch my red ball and listen to my rattle, his mother moved up next to me. He turned to her voice and looked her in the face. She grinned when I spoke, and when he turned to me and followed my face. I felt close enough to the mother by now that I asked her, "Do you have any questions?" She shook her head, but her eyes were glued on me. I said, "Your head says 'no' but your eyes say 'yes!'" Again, she shook her head but kept looking at me. I said, "Your head keeps saying one thing but your eyes another." She nodded slightly. I said, "Shall I ask all these people to leave?" She nodded. When they all left and I asked whether she had any concerns about her beautiful baby, her hand wandered down her baby's belly to his groin. I took off his diaper and was startled to find a huge inguinal hernia. She began to weep. Then, she looked at me carefully and began to tell me that she knew she had ruined her little boy by having sex while she was pregnant. I told her that he wasn't "ruined." We could reduce and fix his hernia. I showed her how this was done and assured her that his masculinity was intact. She continued to weep. Because I was only going to be here one day, would she mind if I called her curer to tell him she was worried, but not tell him why? She said, "He'll never talk to you." I told her I wouldn't expect him to come in here. I would go out to him on the lawn in front of the hospital. She accepted that and called him. I met him outside, told him to comfort her about the baby's hernia but did not mention her reasons for guilt. He said he'd expect her call. I went back in and told her that he'd be ready to help her and that we'd fix the hernia before they left the hospital. Tears flowed, and she reached out to touch me and made a mark of the cross over me.

When I went back to the hospital physicians to tell them of her fears about the hernia and her openness with me, they could hardly believe it. "She never said a word." "Maybe you shouldn't use words," I suggested. "When I used the baby's behavior as my language, she opened up." This visit opened up the Navajo nation to me, and together with colleagues I visited them many times after that. Ned Pablo, a nurse and head of the unit later became trained on the NBAS and began to teach everyone how to use the baby's behavior to communicate with new mothers.

I ended up feeling close to the staff at the hospital and felt they trusted me. I'd become interested in the widespread problem of fetal alcohol syndrome and had developed some approaches to investigate. Among Native Americans, the incidence of fetal alcohol syndrome with severe brain damage, was, at that time, and still is, much higher than for the rest of the United States. There is also an enormously high incidence of less-severe brain damage in the form of fetal alcohol effects, which often goes unrecognized. Victims have mild sensory disorders such as learning disabilities or attentional hyperactive disorders. These can interfere with children's ability to fit into school or their community because their disability got them labeled as "bad." On my visit to this hospital, I began to feel that, if we could identify these children as babies (using my NBAS), we could offer them early intervention and their parents an understanding of them. Otherwise, they were all too likely to fail academically and socially. I preached this plan to Ursula Wilson, who said it was a wonderful idea. We began to construct a proposal and very quickly found faculty at the University of New Mexico to consult with us and help us identify the early signs of fetal alcohol effects.

We designed a study to follow the development of affected children and to offer early intervention. However, when we returned with the money for the study and the consultants as well as for the intervention team, we ran into trouble. We presented our study to the tribal council. They listened attentively, nodding about the problem of alcohol in the community. But our study required identifying the women who drank alcohol, and they refused to allow it. If their women were drinking, it seemed that they didn't want to know about it. "But this affects your next generation of children, and we do know how to help them." "No!" Our study never came to fruition. Ursula Wilson and I were devastated. Later, I wondered whether we would have had more success had we worked more collaboratively with the tribal council from the start.

Ned Pablo, who had trained on my newborn assessment and began to share babies' behavior with new parents, ran into trouble as well. He was not welcome in Navajo newborn hospitals. His work became seen as intrusive in the Navajo community. Other Navajo nurses agreed, as if it were an invasion of the parent-child system. In retrospect I wish that Ursula had been trained in the scale as well. Then our work might have survived.

I have not found this strong resistance in the other Native American tribes that I've gotten to know. I saw that the hierarchy of strong men, and of successful women such as Ursula, was the key to any entry into the Navajo tribe. It was a missed opportunity to have been cut off from the rest of the study and intervention we planned. Newborn Navajo babies were stronger in their reactions than many other native tribes, such as the Maya in southern Mexico. Although as descendants from their Asian ancestors, they had the same genotype, but they were less peaceful as newborns. Many of them were active when they were alert. They cried loudly, demanding attention. They were not as easy to console as the newborns in Mexico that we had seen. It was as if these babies were preparing to fit into Navajo history as one of the most powerful tribes in the Americas.

Greece: Archaeology and Doulas

The mother of two of my patients, Emily Vermeule, was a professor of archaeology at Harvard. She came into my office soon after her second baby was born. Her older child was three years old, and we began to share the issues of sibling rivalry. Then she dropped a bomb. "She'll get to know and take care of Adrian while I'm gone. I'm leaving them to go to the Greek Islands." "What? Leaving a new baby and a three-year-old whom you've just deserted by having a sibling?" "My husband will be here with them." "But that's not enough. You can't just leave your children. They'll suffer, and you'll never forgive yourself." Emily explained that this was the opportunity of a lifetime. The head of archaeology at the University of Athens, Spyros Marinatos, had asked her (and only her) to come help him uncover a major find, from the Mycenaean site that had just been discovered on the island of Thera (colloquially known as Santorini). It had been covered with ash from the volcanic explosion of nearby Crete about 1500 BC. No one knew of it. It was called the "lost Atlantis," although that was probably just to popularize it. She couldn't afford to turn down this opportunity. It would mean being away for an extended period and leaving her children at home with her husband and a babysitter. She felt devastated but helpless. I knew how much it meant to her, as a leading expert on Greek archaeology in this country, to be invited by the Greeks as they uncovered this fabulous find. But my priorities were with her small children and what it might mean to them to be without their mother. "Why can't you take them with you? All of you go as a family. They'd really suffer from not having you, and you'd suffer from leaving them. Take them!" "I can't." "Why not?" "Because there's no doctor on this island and I'd be afraid they'd get sick." "Well, that can be fixed!" "How?" "Take me with you." She looked stunned but recovered enough to say, "Do you mean it?" "I do." "You're on," she said. She even began planning to require that the Museum of Fine Arts, who was sponsoring her, foot my bill as a necessary adjunct to her going.

One of the attractions for me on the island of Thera was to follow midwives, known as *doulas* as they delivered babies at home. We had the opportunity to be in on several deliveries. During delivery, the mother was given tin cans, empty bottles, old shoes. When she had a labor pain, she threw them at her husband who cowered and groaned in a corner of the room. When we offered to relieve him, he said, "No! This is my job!" His participation was so important to her and relieved her of the usual groaning with pain that we saw in delivering mothers elsewhere. A birthing stool was used, a V-shaped stool, eighteen inches high with a hole in the middle. The laboring mother sat astride it at the end, the midwife delivered the baby underneath it. After delivery, the mother was allowed to go to bed. When the baby came, the midwife, who had instructed the mother all through her labor, really delivered her. But I had the luck of helping, and of holding the baby as she slid out. When the baby started breathing, I rushed to show her to the new mother. She turned away toward the wall, saying "not yet." We had been influenced by Marshall Klaus and John Kennell's work and were concerned that unless a mother held and interacted with her newborn at this initial "sensitive" period, she might never attach to her baby. If she had others at home, it seemed even more important that she admire this beautiful, intact baby.

Even her husband, the father who had worked so hard with each labor pain, seemed blasé about holding and admiring the baby. The father was vaguely interested, but he mainly wanted to stroke his wife and to announce the new arrival to all his waiting family. After about thirty minutes of deep breathing and quiet rest, the mother turned toward me and her newborn. She had recovered her own equilibrium. She said quietly, "Now, I'm ready." She examined the baby in detail, smiled, called her by name, and put her to breast to suckle. The baby sucked immediately (no medication to interfere), and the mother and infant were off to a loving start. I had learned a lot: (1) fathers had a major role, (2) childbirth without medication avoids depressing the baby, (3) the initial opportunity to bond with a new baby could be postponed while the mother recovered from labor, and (4) successful breast feeding is enhanced by an alert baby and by the mother's expectation that it would work. When the baby wouldn't suck effectively, the mother would work to alert her. She'd flatten her nipple out by using the fingers to press on her breast, making a flat long triangle of her nipple. When the baby opened her mouth as if to cry, she'd press the nipple way back into her throat. This set off the sucking reflex, which is strong at the back of the throat, and the baby began to nurse. I learned a lot about how to help breast-feeding off to a good start.

We made a study on the infants born at the Mitera, a maternity hospital for unwed mothers, founded in 1958 by Queen Wilhelmina of the Netherlands. We found that there was a significant difference in the behavior of babies whose mothers ate well in the first half of the pregnancy versus the infants of mothers who tried to hide their pregnancy from their fathers and brothers as long as possible by starving themselves. By about five months, they had to leave home and come to Athens. If they came to the Mitera, they were well fed and taken care of for the rest of pregnancy. If they had not been taken care of, their babies would be small for gestational age (SGA) and quite undernourished at birth. These babies whose mothers hadn't eaten well the first half of pregnancy were fragile and hyper-sensitive, crying a great deal and difficult to calm down. These ba-bies were considered unadoptable for months after birth. They were nowhere near as responsive, able to manage alert and sleep states, or to be consoled as the group whose mother had eaten well and been taken care of all through pregnancy. We learned from this study again about the effects of maternal nutrition on the outcome of ba-bies. Since then, we have developed the technology to visualize the brains of newborns whose mothers were not well fed and have con-firmed these findings. Nutrition is a vital precursor to brain develop-ment in utero.

These studies of newborns around the world have taught us that other cultures and their values have many contributions to offer our society. The spectrum of differences in infant behavior or in parents' ways of handling their neonates in these various cultures are valu-able to those caring for parents and babies in the United States. De-spite individual variations within each culture, the differences, from the shy, sensitive children from Asia or southern Mexico, to the more motoric behavior of East African babies points the way to many possible potential changes in our child-care arrangements and our educational system.

We call ourselves a "melting pot," a tolerant nation. But we are not. Children pay a high price for the way we treat families from other cultures. For example, a shy child is less valued in our present society. He is pressed to change, to be a different person. Parents in Asia value a child's high degree of sensitivity to learning materials and to others. Such children gain the feeling of being valuable to the world and to their families. A child who feels validated walks straighter and values himself. The motoric children whom we saw in Kenya, reinforced for their motoric achievements, "learn on their feet." For such children, we could incorporate teaching with physical movement. A child in the United States who is very active is labeled and medicated unnecessarily. Such a child could be valued for his motor achievement, for the intensity of his motor expressions. We could see both the sensitive and the motoric children as being on opposite ends of the spectrum of individual differences and allow for this in our educational system. We are missing so much when we can't welcome many cultures and the differences they bring that can enrich our institutions and society.

FIVE

Bucking the System

en Spock's publication of *Baby and Child Care* in 1946 changed the world of parenting. Before his much-beloved book, parents were supposed to be rigid disciplinarians, often still adhering to the teaching of John Watson, who warned in his 1928 book *Psychological Care of Infant and Child* about the "dangers of too much mother love." "Never hug or kiss them. Never let them sit on your lap," he wrote. Anderson Aldrich in the late 1930s had begun to change the attitudes of pediatricians, pointing out that parents can be cared for and encouraged and helped to understand their children so that they'd do a better job. Spock's book followed and gave parenting back to parents. He described their children, helped them uncover their own feelings, gave them insights into what the child might be thinking, and essentially told them that they were capable of deciding what to do about the child's issues. Following his mentor, D. W. Winnicott, he was the first in the United States to empower parents. As a result, parents began to feel they could make up their own minds about problems that their child might face. He also offered pediatricians insight into the passions that parents brought to their jobs. In practice himself, he modeled to other pediatricians their job of trusting parents to nurture their children's emotional health.

Learning to Like Parents

As a young pediatrician, I began to become aware of my own feelings. I had gone into pediatrics because I liked children. When anything went wrong for them, I automatically felt angry with their parents. They were ready to be blamed, because a passionate parent automatically feels it's her fault when anything goes wrong. But I saw that criticizing a mother resulted only in more guilt and more likelihood of failure in the crises families face. My feelings of blame were an automatic response, which I now call gatekeeping. Every adult who cares about a child is bound to feel competitive with any other adult for that child's well-being. I have seen that when anything goes wrong, any caregiver (pediatrician, nurse, kindergarten teacher) will almost inevitably feel competitive and blame the parent. "If I were that child's parent, she wouldn't be allowed to act like that in public."

Pediatricians are less likely than others to admire parents, until they become parents themselves. Then they begin to understand the passion behind parents' conflicts with their child. But they may still say to a parent, "If you'd only do it this way." A top-down approach from a pediatrician is likely to make parents resent rather than accept ideas that might help. Spock's book modeled an understanding and acceptance of the conflicts all parents face. He certainly helped me realize that if I wanted to help children, I had to accept and help their parents.

I began to see my job as learning to like parents. When I changed and began trusting them, they started to trust themselves.

We were no longer adversaries. We could be a team—and work toward the child's best interests. My patients' parents and I dared to care about each other and to share the child's developmental progress.

As soon as parents could trust me not to be judgmental, I found that they came in with two essential questions at each visit: (1) "How am I doing as a parent?" and (2) "How's my child doing in her development?" I wanted to answer those burning questions for them and realized that to do so I needed to understand child development. There were only a few role models in pediatrics for me to follow.

Milton Senn at Yale and Julius Richmond at Syracuse were outstanding pediatricians who led the way to a respect for parents' feelings. But there was no one who really saw that child development was the language that could unite pediatrics and parents. Urie Bronfenbrenner, a psychologist at Cornell, was one who held out an olive branch to be shared by parents and the child's doctor. A brilliant expert on sociological issues, he predicted the problems still plaguing our present medical system—not enough attention to the prevention of diseases and not valuing the psychological development of the children as part of their ability to resist disease. From his work on the ecology of child development embodied in the family system and in the world at large, I began to see the parent-child relationship as the first bulwark in any successful medical system for families.

Bringing Parents into the Hospital

Close to home I realized that we weren't doing well in promoting mental health at Boston Children's Hospital. In 1967, Dr. Leonard

Cronkhite brought his two children to my office in Cambridge. I was amazed to see a father. Not only did few fathers bring their children for check-ups, but Len was the CEO at Children's, and I knew he was a very busy person. His daughters were wonderful and their check-ups were delightful. One day, as he was ready to go, I commented on the fact that two of the other teaching hospitals (Boston Floating— so named because it was founded as a ship in Boston Harbor offering care and fresh air to the city's children—and Mass General) were instituting parent rooms, with chairs that reclined at night. Parents were being encouraged to stay with their ill, hospitalized children. Children's Hospital's policy, however, allowed parents to visit only from 2–4 p.m. on Saturday afternoon. Children would begin to cry after the visit, would cry all weekend and through Monday. Doctors and nurses would then say, "See, parents are not good for sick children. They upset them. They demand too much of us and are never satisfied. They should just leave their children's care to us and we could get them well and send them home sooner."

But there was beginning to be a surge of literature from research (such as that of Dr. John Lind in Sweden) that demonstrated the cost to children of separation, of the fear of being abandoned, of having to deal by themselves with the pain in hospital care, the loneliness, the fears of being handled and abused by strangers, and, in older children, the fears of the illness and its consequences. Parent presence and parent participation could mitigate all of these. In addition, parents could face their own grief and learn about the illness and how to care for the child before discharge. With the grim work of Harry Harlow showing the devastating effects of separation on baby monkeys and the insights of John Bowlby to back us up, we were convinced that an illness could easily have psychosomatic aftereffects when a child was left alone in the hospital. The chances of parents later hov-

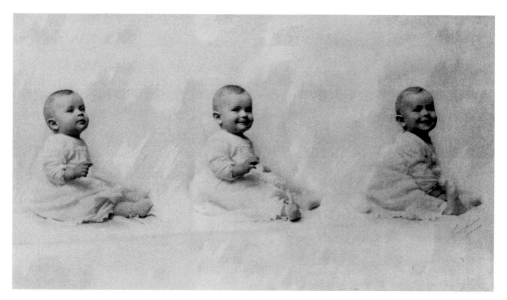

Evolution of a smile at four months

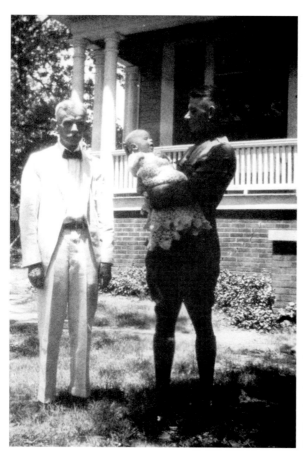

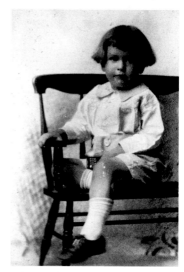

About three years old

With my father, Thomas Berry
Brazelton, and grandfather
William Buchanan Brazelton.
I was nine months old, and my
father, who had been at war, was
seeing me for the first time.

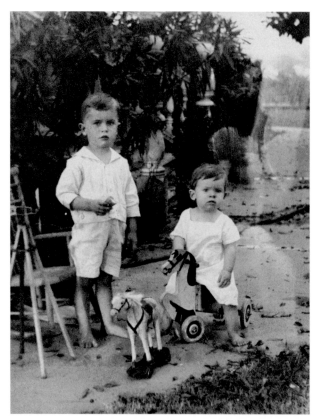

With brother Chuck at my
grandmother's house in Waco

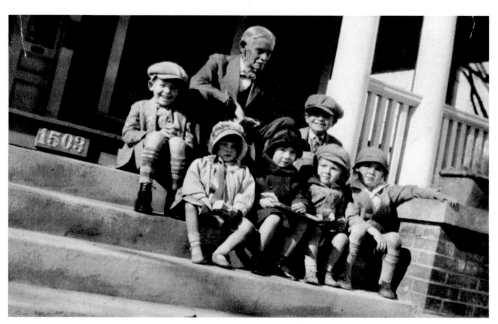

On my grandparents' porch in Waco with my cousins and grandfather. I'm in the top
row on the right.

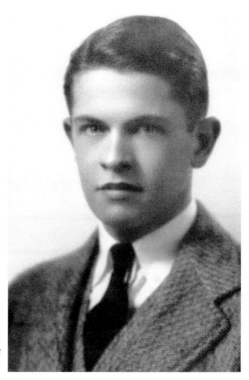

Photo taken for the Princeton Triangle
Club when I was president

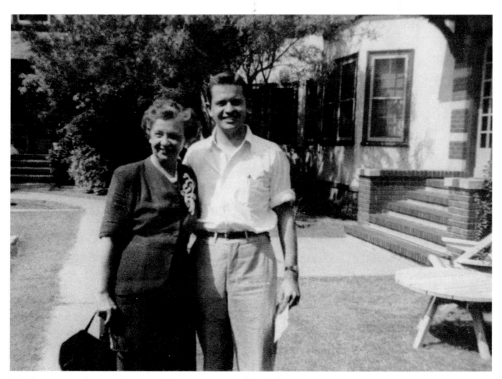

With my mother in Waco after returning from the Navy

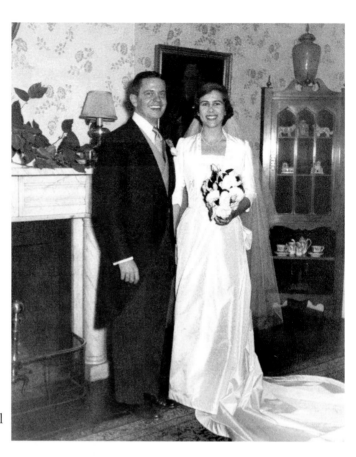

With Christina Lowell
at our wedding

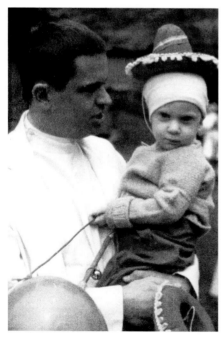

With a young patient at
Massachusetts General Hospital
in 1946

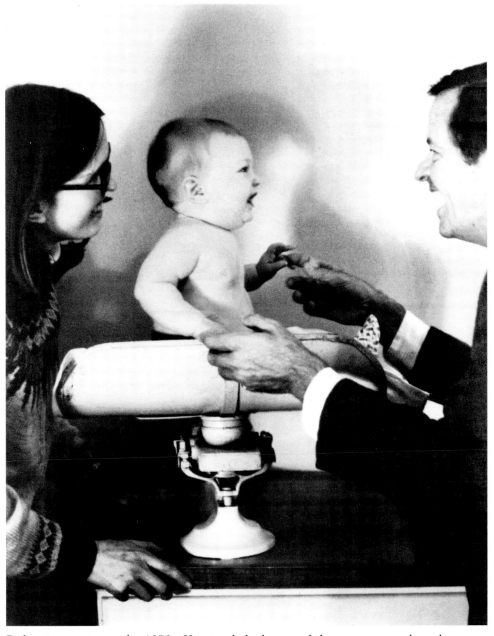

Pediatric practice in the 1970s. Keeping baby happy while on an unsteady scale.
© *Steven Trefonides*

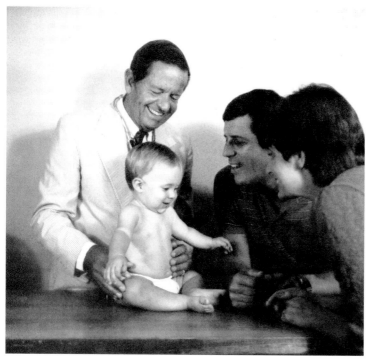

Showing parents how baby at six months sits with hands askew to balance. © *Steven Trefonides*

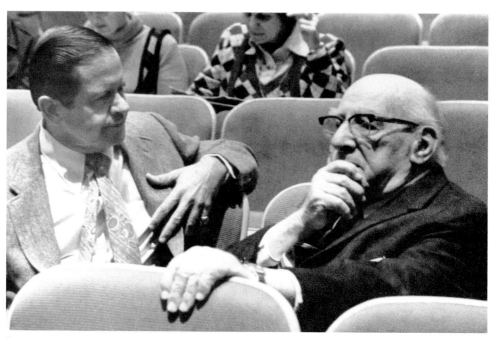

Discussing early deprivation with Rene Spitz at a conference in Denver

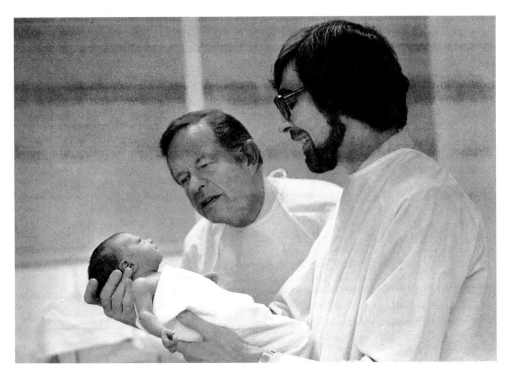

Observing a newborn with Kevin Nugent at Children's Hospital, Boston

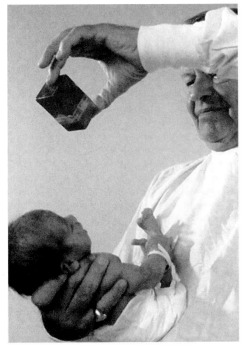

Evaluating an infant's abilities with the Neonatal Behavioral Assessment Scale

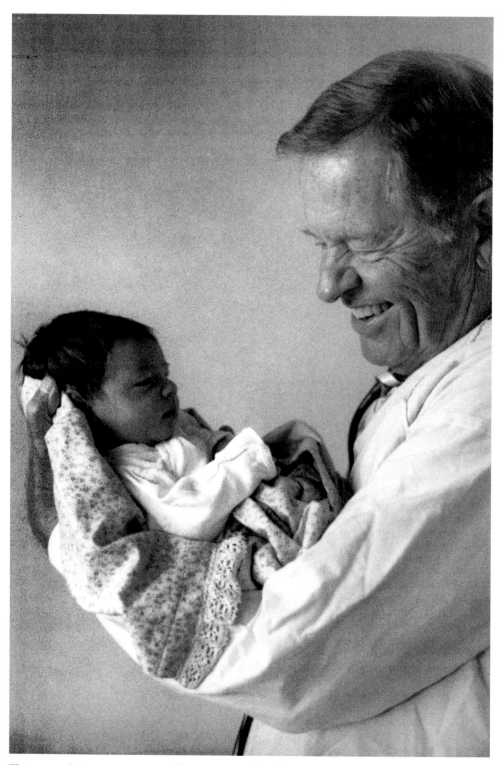

Trying to elicit eye contact with a two-month-old infant. © *Valerie Winckler*

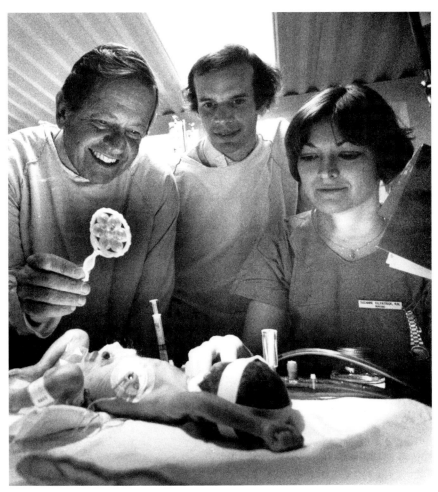

Testing the responses of a premature infant at Children's Hospital with
Peter Gorski and Suzanne Kilpatrick

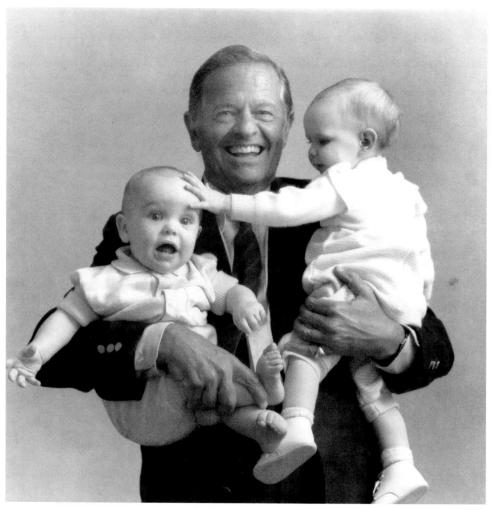

Babies and toddlers are so intensely interested in other children that they can't keep their hands off each other. © *Hornick-Rivlin*

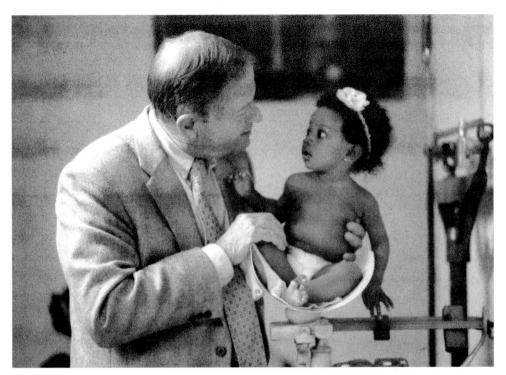

A wary patient. © *Valerie Winckler*

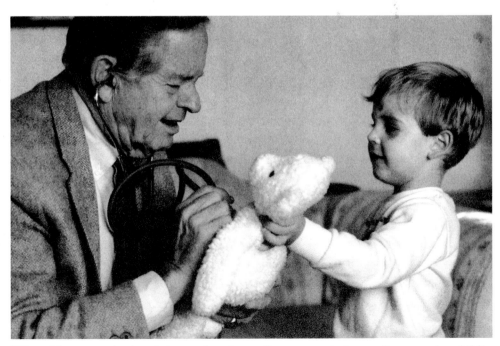

When I listen to the bear's heart first, I usually get permission to listen to the child's.
© *Valerie Winckler*

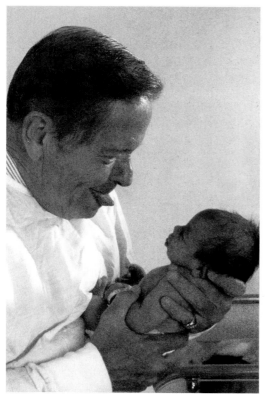

Newborn imitating me

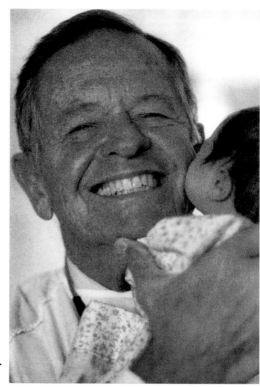

A newborn trying to nurse on my cheek.
© Valerie Winckler

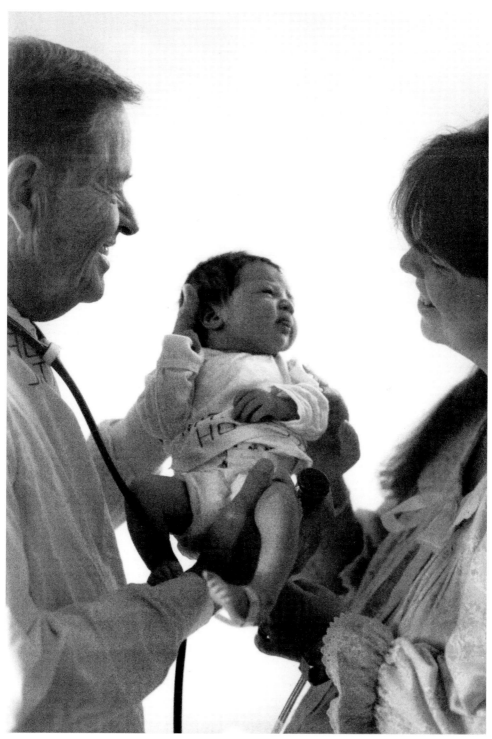

An infant turns first to his mother. © *Valerie Winckler*

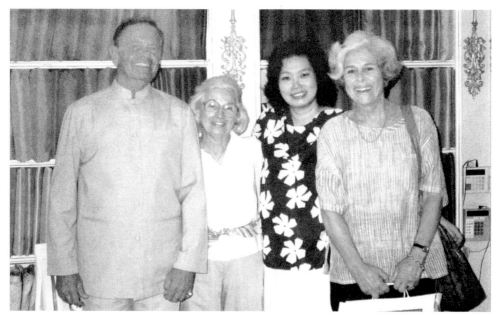

In Japan with Ellen Ross, Nittaya Kotchabhakdi, and Chrissy. *Courtesy of Countway Library, Harvard Medical School*

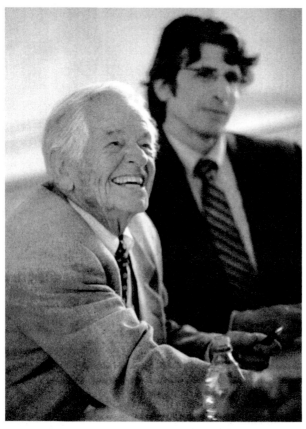

With Joshua Sparrow, coauthor and principal colleague at the Touchpoints Center. *Courtesy of Insieme/Fulvia Farassino*

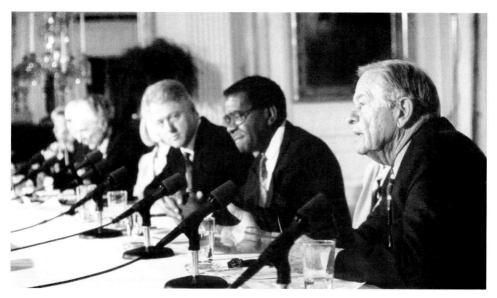

White House conference on early intervention. Hillary Clinton is behind President Clinton and Harry Chugani, MD, is to his left, next to me.

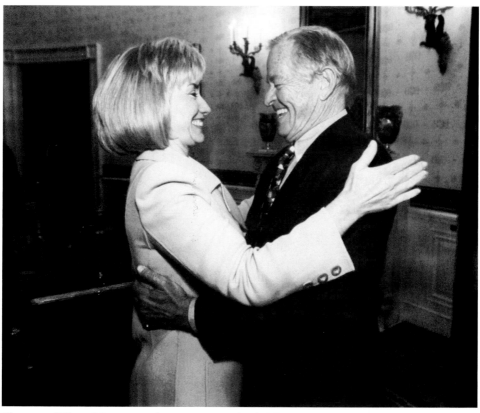

Planning White House conferences on early childhood with Hillary Clinton in 1996

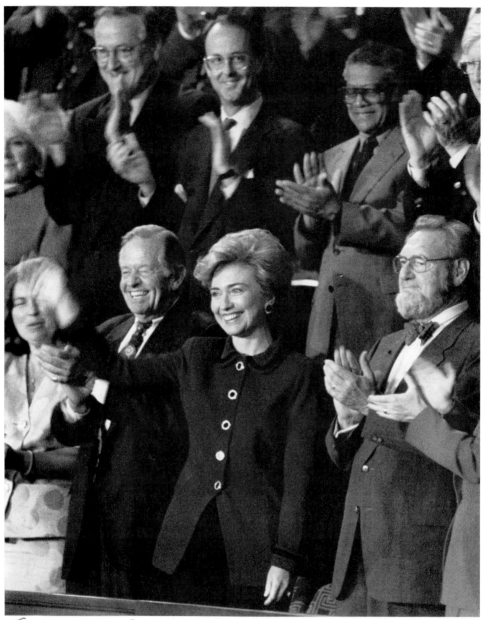

To T. Berry Brazelton with thanks for your support and hopes that we will see our dream of health care for all children realized in 1994. Best wishes, Hillary Rodham Clinton 1993

Applauding President Clinton's speech at the health-care bill debate in 1993.
C. Everett Koop, MD, is to Hillary Clinton's left.

ering, becoming fixed on the child's illness, and thus of ending up with what we came to call vulnerable child syndrome—a child who is overprotected and has internalized the parents' anxieties—was magnified when parents did not understand the illness and especially when they were not aware of the child's resilience and ability to recover. In-hospital parenting was a new and exciting area.

Aware of these studies, I said to Len that I sympathized with parents who did not want their children to go to Children's Hospital unless they had to because of the nature of their illness. Otherwise, they preferred one of the other hospitals with a family approach. Since Children's had superb specialists and was number one in the country for research and treatment, parents often had no choice. I said, "Would you want to abandon your child in a cold, frightening environment just because of an illness?" He listened and said, "Why don't you help us change this practice? I'll back you." Dr. Dane Prugh was head of child psychiatry at the hospital, and he was encouraging, as was Dr. Charles Janeway, head of pediatrics. But I was wary of being put in such a vulnerable, administrative role. I was reluctant to leave my practice and all of my wonderful families. We needed the income as well. I took my ambivalence home to Chrissy. She had wanted me to get involved in academia. She enlisted Jerome Bruner, with whom I was doing research at the time. She and he said, "Come on, you're a big boy, and it's time you took on a bigger role. You can do it." Their encouragement helped me make up my mind. Without abandoning my practice, I decided to take the job of patient care coordinator, working from 10 a.m. (after my 8:30–9:30 a.m. call hour) until 4:30 p.m., returning to see patients from 5 until 7 p.m. It was sure to be a multitasking, busy life, with less time for my family, but Chrissy encouraged it. I became excited about the challenge.

I had no idea how to go about changing a whole hospital's practices. I met with Barbara Patterson, the head of the child activities department and the head of social work at Children's, Elizabeth Maginnis. The latter was a brash, dedicated, strong ally and became a close friend. She said, "Of course you can do it. But don't give up your practice. That will protect you from the destructive competition you'll run into over here."

Muriel Vesey, the head of nursing, was ambivalent but she said she understood what I was talking about and could see it working in the other hospitals. If it didn't overload the nurses, she would be for it. I pointed out to her that a child activities person could work with the child and family and support the nursing role. I got Len Cronkhite to fund a major increase in the number of such psychologically trained "play-ladies"—one for each medical floor. The late Myra Fox led the Child Life Services program for many years.

Liz Maginnis advised me to get all the heads of departments—medicine, cardiology, ENT (ear, nose, and throat), orthopedics, surgery, social work, nursing, physical and occupational therapy, child activities, and admissions—together once a month in order to work together for the change. The heads of departments were willing, largely because their bosses, Drs. Cronkhite and Janeway, told them to come. Other hospitals had already changed, so they knew we had to.

We had meeting after meeting, aired everyone's objections, presented research papers to prove the value of bringing parents into the child's care and to show how other pediatric hospitals were doing it. With Liz's help, we began special rounds on each floor once a week. In these rounds, nurses (and doctors) and others involved would present difficult cases so we could begin to identify the adjustments needed to incorporate parents onto the floors. Over the next few years, the plan began to catch fire, and people began to talk about the change.

Our practice had been to send out a brochure to the parents of all planned admissions, urging them to prepare their child for the separation and admission for surgery. In surveying the parents later, we found that only 15 percent ever read it, even though it contained information about how you could protect your child by preparing him and about the importance to the child of knowing what was going to happen. When we asked them why not, many would finally admit: "I couldn't face it myself." With this knowledge, we decided to offer parents a book called *Curious George Goes to the Hospital* by Margret and H. A. Rey. They were pressed to read it to the child in the admissions office, while a child activities specialist supported them to "face it themselves." Children were significantly more cooperative on the wards after that.

Two of the leaders in the hospital, Alex Nadas, head of cardiology, and Robert Gross, chief of surgery, offered me a chance to study the effects of parent participation on outcomes after cardiac surgery. In this research project, we found that if parents (1) prepared their child for admission (separation, the strange ward, blood tests, examinations), (2) stayed on the ward with the child, (3) accompanied him to the surgery, and (4) stayed with him until the anesthetic took hold, these children not only had a significantly better survival rate but their need for anesthetic, their postoperative recovery, and their hospital stay was significantly reduced. Also, if the parents could be present when he awoke and could nurse him on the ward, playing out his fears and trauma afterward, his recovery was significantly better. This piece of research led to an immediate change all over the hospital. Parents were not only welcomed but were urged to stay twenty-four hours a day with their child. We had done it!

Chairs that could be made into beds for sleepovers were introduced (the parents of my patients gave ten of them). Restructuring and replanning the size of patient rooms began. The whole hospital had a different atmosphere. A parent's cafeteria and waiting room was introduced on each floor.

We found that planned admissions could be further helped if:

- Parents were urged to bring the child in ahead of time to climb in and out of an oxygen tent.
- Admission and post-op play programs were introduced.
- Parents were urged to play "hospital" with their children after they went home.

The actual visits by parents changed. They were taught how to administer meds and how to nurse their children. In the process, they were given support to face their own issues about the child's illness and hospitalization. For the children, the whole experience was different. Of course, they cried more and showed their feelings more openly, but now the medical team could see this as healthy in the long run. The child activities specialists designed therapeutic play for each child and became models for parents who didn't know how to talk with or play with a sick child. The downside of parent presence was that they could be exposed to an insensitive medical team—physicians standing at the bedside to talk about the child as if he were just an illness. Parents often complained about how little they really communicated with medical personnel. Nevertheless, everyone began to recognize the value of the parent presence for the child's recovery.

Sibling visitation did not come about until about twenty years later. On one occasion while it was being considered, some parents came to visit their two-year-old who was dying of a brain tumor. He was fragile, had lost all his hair, and was wasting away. But he tried valiantly to smile and to win the attention of the nurses on Division 27. They adored him. So they kept him in a playpen out by the head nurse's desk. There, they could all talk to him and pat him as they went by. It was a cherished spot and he seemed to love it.

One day, his parents came off the elevator. They went to him to greet and kiss him. He roused briefly to smile half-heartedly at them. But one could feel his reserve, and maybe even his anger, at being left alone in the hospital.

Following the parents, his two older brothers, six and four, slowly came up to him. He began to moan, pulled himself up on his feet, holding onto the playpen railing. He rubbed up against them, feeling their faces. They patted and hugged him. He was obviously in ecstasy. All of the nursery and hospital staff was watching, weeping. This one moment helped make siblings welcome on the wards. No more objections like "they'd bring germs on the floor." Now the hospital is for whole families and they are welcomed, even urged to stay.

After the hospital visiting hours for parents changed, I was asked to do a weekly set of rounds on child development—a teaching experience for house officers, nurses, the therapists on the team, and for Harvard medical students. The rounds became so popular that we had to move into a big room to accommodate as many as fifty personnel.

Listening to the Hospitalized Child

On these rounds, I had the opportunity to demonstrate what the illness meant to each child by using his behavior. How he managed it, how much it cost him, the regression he was going through as he

dealt with his illness. In the demonstration, I would show the medical personnel how to evaluate a child for the different aspects of his
development. These included his emotional development (to whom
he turned—his nurse, his parent, himself, and how important a
"lovey" or his thumb might be as he faced a hospitalized illness), his
cognitive development (how it might show a regression but also allow a window into the child's fears and thoughts; how he used play
as his therapy), his motor development (how the illness affected it
and in turn the other lines of development). We also looked for sensory integration, for if one modality—sight, hearing, touch, or kinesthetic (the sense that detects body position and movement)—were
impaired, the others would automatically be affected.

On the rounds, we also looked at one more important line of
development. Did a child expect to succeed or to fail? Addressing
this question showed us how overwhelmed or how resilient he
might be as he coped with his illness. It was also a window into his
past experiences.

For example, by nine months, we could tell whether a baby expected to succeed or fail by his response to a specific task. When
we'd present an age-appropriate challenge, like making a toy work, a
baby who expected to succeed would puzzle over it, work at it, and,
when he achieved it, he'd look up proudly as if to say, "See, I just did
it! Aren't I great?" But a child who didn't expect to succeed might
get quickly distracted or turn to some activity in which he could succeed, or he might fail deliberately (as with children who came from
overly stressed home situations where no one ever gave them credit
for success). When he failed in the task, you could often see that he
understood it cognitively but he just didn't have the will to struggle
to do it. Then he'd look up cringing as if he expected to be beaten,
reprimanded, or, at best, ignored. At twelve months, the same child

would fall down when he tried to cruise on furniture or walk. Then, he'd look up, cringing. At eighteen months, when he could walk, he'd trip and fall down. When you'd try to see why he fell or what he tripped on, you'd find nothing. When you went to him, he'd cringe and look frightened. These children were already trying to say, "I can't do it. I'm no good." They either came from harsh and unrewarding environments, or they already recognized that they were inadequate to face the tasks you offered. I felt we were sometimes able to see early signs of learning disabilities or ADHD (attentional disorders, sensory integration problems) or maybe even autistic spectrum disorders. We were able to learn so much from careful observation of a child's behavior. I found these rounds to be wonderful ways to teach the staff the different lines of development in small children.

As the change in the hospital rules regarding parents proved itself valuable, we also found that our residency program at Children's was becoming more popular. Word got around the country that Children's Hospital in Boston is interested in the psychological development of children as well as in their illnesses. We were besieged with more and better young intern applicants—especially women.

Ironically, as parental leave began to be recognized in the late 1980s, we needed to face the fact that we treated medical personnel worse than parents. They had no chance to stay at home after a new birth to enhance the new baby's attachment and to understand their new roles as parents. I brought this up with Dr. David Nathan, the chief of pediatrics. He said, "But we can't let a new parent intern off for more than four weeks. After all, other interns and residents have to cover for them and it means raising their workloads." I said, "How many interns and residents at each level do you have?" "Twenty." "Why not increase it to twenty-one at each level so you can have a floating resident who can take up the slack." I reminded him that we were a family-friendly hospital now, professing to believe in the importance of family attachments. Over half of our residents were women who might have new babies. "Shouldn't we be reinforcing their understanding and participation in family attachments? It would be a good investment." David approved and added a new resident at each level. The atmosphere improved again. Not only was parenthood respected but an illness could be covered as well. Resident physicians could take time off without feeling they were burdening their colleagues.

Buoyed by these experiences, in 1973 a group of us had started planning for the future Association for Child Care in Hospitals (ACCH). Eight heads of child activities and child life programs in hospitals around the country came together, led by Mary Brooks from Pittsburgh and others from as far as Montreal. At about the same time in Cleveland, Emma Plank, a wonderful woman who had been a German refugee from the Nazis and now ran the child activities at Rainbow Babies and Children's Hospital, became a vocal advocate for making hospitals sensitive to children's needs. She wrote a classic book, *Working with Children in Hospitals*, which served to change pediatric hospitals in this country.

We gathered this group on the verandah of our home in Barnstable, MA—two men, six women—and worked all day for four days to found the new association. The ACCH began with little funding, and, over the twenty-five years of its existence, never raised any real money. But the annual meetings became popular with nurses, pediatricians, and occupational and physical therapists. Our original idea had been to professionalize the work of child life specialists, but a multidisciplinary approach began to flourish. From about eighty participants in 1974, it grew to several hundred by the 1980s. John Kennell from Case Western Reserve, Sprague Hazard from Harvard, Kyle Pruett from Yale, and Stan Friedman from Albert Einstein Hospital supported our efforts.

In the 1990s, the Child Life Council, which was a professional organization for child life specialists, began to take over. By the nineties, it had supplanted ACCH and served the purpose of professionalizing all of the workers, our original goal. This mission appears on their website today: "Child life programs in health care settings promote optimum development of children and their families, to maintain normal living patterns and to minimize psychological trauma." Today, child life professionals organize play that is both therapeutic and entertaining and prepare children for and help children during medical tests and procedures. They also support families during hospitalization or challenging events. They work in a variety of health care facilities, maintaining a philosophy of family-centered care.

Bringing Child Development into Pediatrics

In the typical short pediatric checkup of the 1960s and '70s, a doctor could only weigh, measure, and give a cursory exam to the child. There was little time or attention for the questions all parents brought: "Should I let her cry?" "When should he start to crawl?" Nevertheless, as I mentioned, what all parents wanted to know was "How am I doing as a parent? How is my child doing?" When these questions weren't answered, everyone lost—the parent, the child, and the pediatrician. When I had made a point to answer, I had a very different experience. Listening to parents' questions about the psychological side of development gives the pediatrician a view of the child as a person, not just a set of illnesses and medical problems.

The child's development also gives parent and pediatrician a common language in which to connect.

During this same time, our pediatric medical system was becoming increasingly sophisticated: heart surgery, antibiotics, early neurological diagnosis. All this was costly and demanded a substructure of good clinical medicine for early diagnosis and follow-up. Mental disorders, the most costly health problems of all to society, were also beginning to be more recognized by the late 1960s. Less deep-seated mental disorders could be prevented by early intervention. Children with a range of developmental disabilities would profit from early diagnosis and intervention. We had become aware of the fact that even autism, one of the most severe mental disorders, could benefit from early diagnosis and intervention.

Many of us in pediatrics knew that we had our hands on a gold mine of opportunities to diagnose and predict and intervene to enhance mental health and development. But the leading medical organizations—the American Medical Association, the American Academy of Pediatrics (AAP), and the Research Society, were all aimed at supporting advances in physical disorders. There were no associations primarily paying attention to child development and the prevention of mental illness. Psychiatric organizations focused on psychopathology, on problems after the fact. Yet we knew that pediatricians could play major roles in the prevention of mental disorders. My own research and practice was teaching me to fight for this opportunity.

Such leaders as Anderson Aldrich, Ben Spock, Milton Senn, Julius Richmond, and Stan Friedman were the models on which I depended for the development of my own career. I knew I wanted to identify children's problems early. My practice in Cambridge helped me develop approaches to help parents prevent deviations in their child's development. I had the opportunity to discuss them with colleagues who were trained in psychiatry as well as pediatrics—such as Norman Sherry, Sprague Hazard, Joel Alpert, Dane Prugh, and Helen Glaser. We felt that the lack of support from our national associations was a critical mistake. We wanted to generate interest in this area of prevention, but no one at these organizations seemed to listen.

Having been active in the section on child development of the AAP, I gained a voice. I was also elected to a special organization of researchers and academicians, the Society for Pediatric Research (SPR) because of my publications on early assessment and infant development. Bob Haggerty, professor of pediatrics in Rochester, New York, and I asked for an SPR symposium as part of the annual meetings of the AAP to address the opportunity to prevent mental illness. The meeting planners predicted that such a symposium would not be able to compete with symposia on cardiac and pulmonary medicine and other rapidly developing research on physical disorders. It took us six years to get a slot. When we finally succeeded, more than three hundred pediatricians attended, standing around the walls of our packed room. It turned out to be the most popular symposium of the meeting. Clearly, pediatricians were hungry for ideas about mental health issues. We made our point, and this segment of both the SPR and of the AAP began to rise to a proper place in pediatric thinking. We established a section on child development within the SPR. The Society for Developmental and Behavioral Pediatrics (SDBP, now with a membership of eight to nine hundred clinicians and researchers) is a result of these efforts.

In 1970, while we were trying to generate interest in child de-velopment as an addition to pediatric teaching and in hospital res-idency, I was made chair of the section on child development in the AAP. It was a wonderful opportunity to get to know those in pediatrics who were as passionate as I was to push the role of pedi-atricians in dealing with the roots of mental health disorders as well as advocating for early intervention for children with special needs. As a section, we met once a year at the academy meetings. Our progress was slow. I was too naive about the politics involved to obtain the support we needed to change the training of pediatri-cians and the thinking of pediatric clinicians. Had I been more so-phisticated, we might have achieved our goals sooner.

We did find ways, however, to get attention. Sprague Hazard and I went to Chicago to a board meeting in the offices of the AAP. We were trying to enlist the board of directors to back preventative men-tal health training. We hoped for a chance to speak at their meeting.

When it became clear that we would not be invited to speak, Sprague and I sat down on the floor on opposite sides of the big door to the boardroom. We stretched out our legs, blocking entry. As each famous professor of pediatrics from around the country came to enter the meeting, they had to step over us. Each one, looking down at us, would say, "What in the world are you two doing?" We said, "We're trying to get your attention." Once we had it, they asked what we wanted. "We want a division of develop-mental pediatrics for training young pediatricians." Most of them first harrumphed. A few of them looked as if they were starting to say, "What is child development?" but they choked it back. We could see that they couldn't make a connection to their kind of pe-diatrics, and we anticipated that very little would happen. Preventive pediatrics still got little attention, and prevention of mental disorders was a long way away from AAP priorities.

Yet I knew that what we were fighting for was sound. Gradually, I began to be invited to lecture on these issues at Cornell, Yale, and at Boston University School of Social Work, where I was made an adjunct professor. By 1976, I was beginning to receive wonderful support and a chance to advocate for my ideas. I received the Lula Lubchenco award from the University of Colorado in Denver. (She was the avant-garde neonatologist mentioned in Chapter 3.) In 1977, I became visiting professor at Rochester with Bob Haggerty and then visiting professor at the University of Hawaii in 1978.

Although the AAP eventually recognized me and in 1983 gave me the C. Anderson Aldrich Award—their highest award—they still did not recognize the kind of work I was doing. In the 1980s I had started a fellowship in behavioral and developmental pediatrics at Children's Hospital that was becoming recognized and had a waiting list of pediatricians. Morris Green and Bob Haggerty had published an influential textbook on clinical and preventive pediatrics that established the theoretical foundation for our efforts. But we still couldn't get the academy to pay attention to our requests to make training in child development and preventive pediatrics part of medical school and residency.

By that time, however, I became worn out trying at the AAP level. My energies were going into Zero to Three: National Center for Infants, Toddlers, and Families and into the Society for Research in Child Development (SRCD). I had left the fight at the AAP to Morris and Bob and to Stan Friedman and Joel Alpert. After they established and fueled the SDBP, that group gave me their founder's award. They have kept up the pressure on the AAP.

At the age of fifty-eight, as these ideas gained traction, I was promoted to become clinical professor of pediatrics at Harvard and Children's Hospital. The clinical track is one reserved for clinicians who contribute to teaching and who do research but do not run a department. I was delighted and grateful to Dr. David Nathan, head of our department at Children's.

I felt that Children's should have a chair in child development to convince pediatricians all over the country to use the behavioral changes in children as they develop as a language to reach parents. It was not until 1995 that this happened and a Brazelton Chair in Pediatrics was established at the Harvard Medical School. Because of our success at Harvard and Children's Hospital, the AAP began to recommend what we had learned be incorporated into the training of pediatricians all over the country. Pediatricians became able to answer the questions parents brought about child and family development. Pediatricians and children's hospitals are following our lead all over the country. The AAP has even launched the Bright Futures program, providing materials on children's behavior for pediatricians and other health providers. Today, however, with the transition to HMOs and managed care and the loss of power of our medical societies, the ability of pediatricians to take the time with parents needed to form a partnership and prevent problems is again threatened.

Training Fellows in Child Development

As we gathered success in changing the atmosphere at Children's Hospital, Dr. Janeway suggested that I begin to train other pediatricians. He thought we ought to look for funding to develop a fellowship in behavioral and developmental pediatrics—a two-year opportunity for young pediatricians after they finish their residencies in general pediatrics. Margaret Mahoney, one of the vice presidents at Commonwealth Fund, was interested. She funded training for four pediatricians a year. It was the Cadillac model and I couldn't believe it.

In 1970 we started the Child Development Unit at Children's Hospital. Ed Tronick, a psychologist with whom I'd worked while doing research with Jerome Bruner, came over to help run our research. At the Child Development Unit, he was trained in the NBAS, and he was interested in the face-to-face research that I had started in Bruner's group with Barbara Koslowski and Mary Main (who later helped to perfect Mary Ainsworth's attachment work).

Ed and I took on the job of trying to train pediatricians in child development while pursuing our research. We had support from Julius Richmond, who was now at Judge Baker Children's Center and at Harvard. He'd always wanted to see this kind of training done and had tried it in CCNY before he came to Harvard. Milton Senn at Yale and Bob Haggerty in Rochester were other role models who had trained pediatricians at a fellowship level in behavioral pediatrics. Our fellows came from all over the country, a superb bunch of people. We knew very little about how to train or how to engage these doctors, who were already well trained in children's diseases, but we knew they knew little about the whole child or about parenting. Our first taker was a star, Daniel Rosenn, a pediatrician who had been working with the Navajos in Arizona. His wife, Barbara, had designed a booklet for Navajo children and had worked in a Navajo child-care center while Dan was completing his training in Shiprock. Dan and Ed and I designed the training that first year, the basics of which lasted for twenty years.

The most striking and innovative part of the training was a half day in which we all simply unloaded with one another our problems with patients and with ourselves. We talked about why we went into pediatrics, what was missing, what frustrated us in our training. It was a spectacular opportunity for all of us to reach into our own past, our own biases, and our own conflicts and to become more self-aware. Nowadays, it is called reflective supervision or reflective practice, and it became the highlight of our training. We would unload ideas and experiences with such passion and enthusiasm that we have never forgotten some of the resulting insights.

As an example, we asked why we didn't include fathers in taking a child's history when we have both parents in our office. We are much too likely to turn to the mother, to ask her all the questions, almost ignoring the father. We wondered why this should be. As we talked, many answers emerged:

(1) "We've been trained to talk to one person and to relate to one—it is very hard to try to include two at the same time."
(2) "Fathers naturally retreat and turn over the answering to their wives, so we don't get much response from them."
(3) "Mothers are more important to children's development than fathers."

Finally, our women trainees admitted that they felt a bit threatened when they got too close in questioning fathers. Then the male trainees admitted that they found themselves on shaky ground if they got too close to another male. All of this made us aware of how many layers of biases were involved in our behavior and how they interfered with our work as a result. In those valuable sessions, we took apart each aspect of practice and the relationships we made with our patients, their parents, and the communities.

We also had a behavioral assessment clinic, which was very productive. The room had a one-way mirror, behind which we could all
sit while one of us interviewed a patient. In that way, we could share
ideas, observations, and criticisms. We discussed difficult patients
and learned from each other. We knew it was important to make fellows aware of their personal history (the ghosts from their own
nursery) and biases. As a result, we got to know each other well.

I loved the training setup we were able to establish, developing
it together. Ed Tronick, Heidi Als, Barry Lester, and Elizabeth
Maury were all critical as psychologist members of the training
team. Several people joined the clinic after the fellowship ended:
Kate Buttenweiser as a social worker, Connie Tagiuri as a child psychiatrist, and Ann Stadtler as a pediatric nurse practitioner.

The fellows spent a day in each of two child-care situations, one
in Brookline (mostly white middle class) and one in Roxbury (African American and poor). They were stunned by the cultural differences, and the experience gave them an opportunity to understand
and discuss them. In the white middle-class day care, each occasion
for discipline was treated as an opportunity—for choices, for reflecting. My fellows all related to that "wonderful day care!" Then, in
Roxbury, discipline was stricter—usually quick and firm. The caregiver would even shout "Stop!" without any explanation. The fellows came back from such an experience saying, "The teachers are
so mean. They don't give children any reason for their discipline."
I pointed out that maybe there were good reasons. Two-year-olds
in Roxbury had to be aware of their surroundings, which were full of
dangers that required stern warnings. We discussed the reasons why
the teachers might seem abrupt and use one-word commands for
discipline. If a situation seemed dangerous, a parent or teacher

might feel there was little time to lay out the reasons for decision making. I think my fellows began to see the differences in the environment of these cultures that could lead to significant differences in how adults deal with children. Although it didn't teach children about how and when to stop themselves, which might be a more optimal goal, it taught children that when an adult spoke with authority in order to protect them, it needed to be taken seriously. The chance to use each disciplinary episode for teaching them to make their own choices was a luxury families could not afford.

Our clinic at Children's was a major teaching opportunity. Once weekly, using three rooms (two for interviews, one for observation), all of us could watch through the one-way glass without intruding on the physician during his relational and diagnostic work. There was a break in the middle of the interview in which the fellow could come behind the screen to get advice and support, to evaluate the diagnostic information that had emerged, and to flesh out what was necessary to secure a full diagnosis. The interviews involved small children or infants whose parents were crying for help. As opposed to other clinics, we were able to follow these families over time. Fellows could learn how to observe behavior, how to collect pertinent history, and how to create relationships that were therapeutic as well as diagnostic. Meanwhile, we had the resources of the Children's Hospital for referral whenever necessary. We all learned the importance of a long-enough interview to collect data, observe, and make relationships. Having the backup of different disciplines was invaluable in giving the young trainees the idea of teamwork, of different perspectives and techniques in caring for families.

Over the years, we trained about sixty pediatricians and a number of nurse practitioners in our two-year fellowship. They have spread out all over the country. Many are professors of pediatrics now, heads of pediatric departments, and in private practice. At least four, including Dan Rosenn, went into child psychiatry and made their marks there. All are versed in child development and have earned the title behavioral developmental specialist. It has now become a specialty within pediatrics. The American Academy of Pediatrics also now demands training in child development from every candidate for AAP certification.

When we began to train nurse practitioners, it seemed to me that they were already trained to foster relationships with parents and their knowledge of child development was way ahead of pediatricians. I felt it would be a good chance for pediatricians and nurses to learn to work together as teams. It was.

At first, the pediatricians would all sit together, as would the nurses. Gradually, as we shared past experiences on Monday afternoons, these barriers began to break down. They began to talk with each other. They began to formulate ways that nurses and physicians could become a team to work together. In the process, we all realized how rigid these walls of professionalization had come to be. Biases operate only if you aren't aware of them. If you become aware of them as biases rather than "the way you operate," they no longer control your behavior—you have a choice. We all learned from this about the barriers different disciplines use to defend their territory. Now, with pediatric care limited by managed-care insurance regulations, teamwork is all the more critical to the kind of care we want to give children.

I learned how much nurses' training had fitted them for the role of respecting and nurturing young families. Pediatricians have been trained for authoritative, top-down roles. Nurses are more likely to be trained to listen, to care, to work with families. It was a real boost to our training of developmentalists to have this point of view firmly integrated into our approach.

In training these fellows, we laid out stages of development to help them understand the likely concerns of parents. My practice was leading me to develop the concepts that I later turned into "Touchpoints" (see Chapter 6).

The insights that I wanted to incorporate into the training came directly from my practice:

(1) The parents are to be considered the experts in their own child's development—behavioral, psychological, and physical development, as well as temperament. No one knows more than the mother and father, and trying to teach them what to do is an ineffective way to help them. They will learn from within—from feeling what is right and what is wrong for their own child.

(2) Training needs to change from a model of watching only for disease and disability to one of highlighting the good things parents are doing with their child. Medical school trains us to look for negatives.

(3) We must value passion wherever it is found—negative can be turned into positive passion. This was a point that needed explanation when a young doctor encountered desperate parents. I often used an experience I'd had in the grocery store with a two-year-old who was taking everything off the shelves. His mother tried to stop him— whereupon he threw a temper tantrum. She was scolding and slapping him. Though I felt like holding her arms to stop her, I said, "Isn't it tough bringing a two-year-old to the grocery store?" She nodded and knelt down to begin

to cry. Her two-year-old climbed up into her lap. Her passionate attempt to make her toddler behave turned into positive nurturing.

(4) A team is essential to provide the backup that stressed parents need. The pediatrician is only one member of this team, though a vital one. We need nurses, therapists, the people at the front desk, everyone in the clinic or hospital to be ready to back up families who need help.

(5) Cultural insights are necessary to understand what families and children are trying to achieve as they face assimilation into the dominant culture.

(6) Using these concepts could lead to powerful and continuing relationships between parents and their pediatricians. Each period of crisis gives the pediatrician an opportunity to understand and become closer to parents.

In other parts of our research that we introduced into our training program, we identified the four earliest stages of attachment behavior between the parents and infants described in Chapter 3. Watching the pattern of attention-withdrawal-attention-withdrawal between mothers and their babies provided us with an opportunity to understand how a parent learns how to relate to and capture the infant's attention and responses in the first four months. This research was instituted when I was at Jerome Bruner's and became the basis for observing and diagnosing the behavior and the rhythmic exchange seen in a clinical office setting. Progress through the stages could be derailed or slowed when the parent was depressed or not attached or if the infant were delayed or not responsive. Smiling, vocalizing, motor behavior all fit into these stages. The violation of these natural interactions introduced by Ed Tronick in his "still face" experiment mentioned earlier, helped prove the depth of the attachment.

Our research on attachment attracted attention. In the late seventies, I was asked to serve on committees of the SRCD. Through this association, I worked with luminaries—Mary Ainsworth, Harriet Rheingold, Arnold Sameroff, Ed Zigler, Urie Bronfenbrenner, Alicia Lieberman, Stanley Greenspan, Reginald Lourie, Kathryn Barnard, Bob Emde, Mickey (Marilyn) Segal, and many, many others. Many of these colleagues became good friends. Later I became president of SRCD—a distinguished but frightening role. As president and representing the clinical side of child development, I felt an enormous responsibility to encourage research on the part of the pediatricians in the field. Such research as we have seen has led to changing many aspects of the system: pediatric office visits, the care of hospitalized children, premature babies, and children who may potentially have special needs, and the training of pediatricians and nurses.

SIX

Touchpoints

A Powerful Relationship

The parents of my patients over the years I was in practice in Cambridge (about twenty-five thousand of them) brought me new little nuggets of insight every time they came for a checkup. Each was like a thank you for our relationship, which had grown to mean a great deal to them, to the child, and to me. I had worked hard to get to know them and help them with each child, and they knew and appreciated it. My first chance to get to know them was before delivery, demonstrating to them that the fetus would pay attention to a rattle or their voices even in the uterus. After the delivery, sharing the baby's behavior with them using my NBAS deepened our bond. Then, after the end of the first year and a half, after inoculations had been completed and the toddler was terrified of me, I made a huge effort to win him back. I insisted that the parent bring in the child four times without charge toward the end of the second year. Each visit was just to become acquainted again and nothing else would be done.

First visit—Parent and child were asked to sit in my waiting room. I'd offer the child a toy or a lollipop. If the child would accept it, that was all.

Second visit—To receive the toy, the child must come off the parent's lap and across the room.

Third visit—He must come around the corner to accept it. I would wear my stethoscope and have my otoscope in hand.

Fourth visit—He would have to come into my office with his mother or father following him to accept my present. Then he had to sit in his parent's lap, and I'd examine his parent's heart and chest first, then his if he was no longer afraid of me. If he would let me, I'd ask him to open his mouth and examine his throat and even look in his ears.

By then, children were usually thrilled to come to my office and were no longer afraid to let me examine them. After all four visits, I don't remember any child who screamed when coming to my office.

Parents were grateful for these efforts to get their child used to me and were eager to share information about their child. I heard how a child worked to learn a new step in development, how much he struggled, how much the parent participated, and how rewarding it was when he finally accomplished it. I came to realize that there were certain times in each child's development when he fell apart, became irritable, and wouldn't eat or sleep. The parent fell apart too, became anxious, and inevitably called me for help. "Is he teething?" "Why won't she eat?" "How do I get him to sleep longer than two hours a night?" These vulnerable times appeared to be common to all the families. I began to realize that they represented the child's struggle just before a new burst in development, such as taking a first step or beginning to speak. When the child regressed and fell apart, he was gathering steam for the next spurt. If I could reassure parents that this was normal and that they needed to let the child struggle on his own, then when he made that next spurt it would be twice as exciting, for he'd be able to feel that he did it himself. Each of these times were opportunities for the parents to get to know the child better, to understand their role with him better, and for me to connect with the parents. I wrote several papers in the 1980s and '90s about what I then called anticipatory guidance.

A Universal Map

Starting in the 1970s my colleagues and I at Children's Hospital began to lay out a map of behavioral and emotional development identifying these predictable times, which I began to call Touchpoints. Since then it has been refined by years of research at Children's and other sites around the world. The same patterns have been identified in other cultures. Six Touchpoints occur within the first year, three or four in the second, and two or three in subsequent years.

The map is designed to reassure parents that regressions lead to predictable spurts in development and that they can navigate them with the resources they can find within themselves, their communities, and their cultures. Unlike yardsticks of physical development (the heights, for instance, that parents take such pride in marking off on door frames), this map has many dimensions. Emotional, behavioral, motor, and language development each occurs at its own pace, but they also affect each other. A child's advances in any one of these areas are preceded by temporary backslides, or regressions, in the same area or another. The cost of each new achievement, in crankiness, negativity, and stress, can temporarily disrupt the child's progress—and the whole family's stability. Yet each of these disruptions also offers parents a chance to reflect, consider a change in direction, and grow along with the child.

One of the gifts from this map is the opportunity for parents to observe with the pediatrician or health-care provider the way the expensive demands of a child's developing nervous system are fueled. There are two sources. One is the internal feedback system described by Robert White and Jean Piaget, seen in any child as she works at a task. When she achieves it she feels a sense of self-worth. "I just did it! I did it myself!" Fuel is also provided externally by parents who applaud the achievement. These two kinds of feedback encourage a child's development.

The concept of Touchpoints is a theory of the forces for change that drive a child's development. Though expressed differently in different cultures, they are probably universal because they are for the most part driven by predictable sequences of brain development, especially in the first three years of life. By showing parents these challenging but exciting landmarks, we can give them the confidence that comes from knowing that their child's development is following common patterns and is progressing in a healthy way. The Touchpoints become a window through which parents can view the great energy that fuels their child's learning. Each step accomplished leads to a new sense of readiness for the next. When seen as natural and predictable, these periods of regressive behavior are opportunities for parents to understand the child more deeply and to support her growth, rather than to become locked into a struggle. A child's particular strengths and vulnerabilities, as well as temperament and coping style, all come to the surface at such a time. We published papers on this concept, and in 1992 I wrote a book called *Touchpoints* for parents.

A Dutch ethnologist, Frans Plooij, told me that he had observed a similar pattern of growth spurts and regressions in chimpanzee infants and mothers! "Why do you sound so surprised?" he asked, reminding me that 98 percent of our genome is shared. Unlike humans, the chimp mothers don't call their pediatricians when their infants regressed. But they often appear to predict these changes, isolating their babies from the pack before the male chimps became annoyed with the intensified crying and clinging. After reading *Touchpoints*, scientists from a variety of fields assured me that many kinds of important changes in nature unfold in this way, with disorganization an inevitable precursor for reorganization at a new and more complex level.

Touchpoints Training

In the 1990s we began to see that the Touchpoints model would be useful in training professionals who care for mothers and babies. We assembled a team from Children's Hospital, Harvard Medical School, and the Harvard Graduate School of Education to design a program for teaching about the model. In 1995 we had our first pilot training in Boston of professionals from three community sites: in California, Indiana, and South Carolina. Each year more sites have been added. There are now 180 Touchpoint sites. These are multidisciplinary sites made up of nurses, physicians, therapists, early education teachers, and child-care workers. They come from communities that are ready for change. We offer them a new approach, using relationships as the basis of their work with parents.

Our model has certain unique aspects:

1. It is a positive model. We value parents' strengths and their passions and see them as the experts, rather than looking for their failures, their mistakes.
2. It is a collaborative model in which providers work with parents as a team. They must face their biases in order to collaborate.
3. It is a developmental model in which the behavior and the development of the child becomes the language between providers and parents. Understanding the predictable disorganization and anxiety that accompanies each regression just before a spurt in development allows the provider to join the parent at each of these times of vulnerability.
4. The model is based on a systems theory instead of a stimuli-response model. The family is a system in which each member is in balance with the other members. If a stress to the system is presented, each member will react in order to return to homeostasis. If providers want to assess whether the reaction is positive or negative, they must learn a great deal about the family—their culture, their past experience, their passion, their values.

Our model requires that parents be involved from the first—the earlier we can start, the more significant will be the results. Also, as we worked with the dedicated professionals of the many communities in our training, we needed to reassure them that Touchpoints was not a program that told them what to do but offered insights to add to what they were already doing.

The Touchpoints model has also been applied in programs aiming to prevent child abuse. When we began, this was a niche in preventive programs that was not yet being filled. Zero to Three in Washington, DC, did good work in this area once abuse problems had been identified. We thought that using the children's development to work with the parents might *prevent* problems. Outreach programs around the country sought to reach and work with troubled parents. We wanted to reach them *before* they were troubled. At the times when children regressed to gather steam for a new developmental spurt, parents are put under greater stress. We have found four Touchpoints in the first two years when we believe we can *prevent* child abuse by redoubling our supports, rather than intervening after abuse has happened. Parents at risk of abusing their children who feel supported and safe are more likely to turn to a caregiver for the help they need rather than abusing the child.

Many of the insights that now inform the Touchpoints work grew from the unusual way we developed the training curriculum at the beginning. Psychologist Ed Tronick, early educator John Hornstein, nurse practitioner Ann Stadtler, with me as the MD, and others developed a theoretical case. We created the story of a patient named Shelley and her newborn, her significant other, and her mother. At each stage, we described their problems. First I would say what I would have done to help them. Each of the others would criticize my approach, ask my reasons for it, and we'd examine my motives, the parents' responses, and the child's behavior. We would discuss why we'd do what we did, and these ideas led us to devise approaches to each of the Touchpoints. We learned so much and put it all together into a curriculum designed to train caregivers as they helped parents face each stage (Touchpoint) in their child's development. We criticized and argued with each other to refine each step in the curriculum and had a great time in the process. We then gathered eight very experienced pediatric nurses and two pediatricians to test this curriculum with us. Again, we asked for feedback and criticism that helped us further refine our program.

Later we developed "train the trainers" courses to allow the program to grow. Trainees who become trainers return to their communities and train many hundreds of professionals in all the disciplines that serve infants, children, and their families.

A Broadening Outreach

The Brazelton Touchpoints Center has worked with nonprofit and government organizations, early childhood departments of universities and colleges, pediatric residency programs, tribal Head Start programs, health centers, schools of nursing, and numerous quality improvement programs in early childhood education. Our Brazelton Touchpoints model has been embraced by tens of thousands of providers of early care and education, health care, and early intervention, reaching millions of families across the country.

Our experiences have led us to believe that the health and prosperity of a community can best be measured by its commitment to give all children the opportunity to thrive, regardless of socioeconomic, family, or cultural differences. One of our goals for the program is thus for the trainers who go back to their communities to train not just the child health providers but also the telephone operators, bus drivers, greeters at the hospital, and child-care sites. When everyone sees the importance of parents as the experts, a positive atmosphere is amplified.

Trainers must also face the inevitable competitive feelings they will have with other professionals as they work to practice our model. Perhaps most important among those who share the child with parents today are child-care providers in day care and nursery school. Most parents must place their babies and toddlers in outside care. Child-care workers are bound to compete with parents. If they express a judgmental attitude, parents won't feel welcome at the child-care site. The providers need to know how parents grieve about sharing their child at the center. I believe that parents defend themselves from grief in three ways: (1) denial—of most of their feelings, (2) projection—they project any problems onto everyone else so they don't need to blame themselves, and (3) detachment—which can be destructive to them and the child.

The centers that have sent providers to our trainings often hear about our model at our "roadshows" (the seminars for professionals and parents we do around the country), as well as by word of mouth from other participants. At the roadshows we lay out the requirements for training. Communities choose a multidisciplinary team to attend our week of training. We learned, however, that one week of training is not enough to absorb our model and that the teams in these communities need to be followed up.

When I discuss the concept of Touchpoints with parents and describe the role a pediatrician, nurse practitioner, or family physician can play in interpreting the regressions and spurts of development with parents, many tell me that their own doctors focus only on assessing physical growth and dealing with illness. Parents often feel that their doctors do not want to answer their questions, when sometimes they may not know how. Though progress has been made, pediatric training is still based largely on the medical model—with its emphasis on tests, treatments, and disease—and still often fails to help doctors learn to identify a child's emotional and behavioral development. Doctors also don't often receive the training they deserve to learn how to collaborate with families and build strong therapeutic relationships. "Managed" care makes this more difficult when it treats doctors as technicians who are too costly to deploy except in limited roles in which skills that only they possess are required. As a result of efforts to reduce the art of medicine to algorithms, doctors are taught to teach and to tell, instead of to listen, and to make up for lack of time with brochures that parents are unlikely to read. This may save time in the short term, but families' most important concerns and questions may be pushed aside.

The power of the therapeutic relationship has been demonstrated by medical research over and over. With its loss, the quality of health care is gravely compromised. If the costs of neglected prevention, missed diagnoses, and bad outcomes are factored in, the magnitude of this lost opportunity is even more daunting. Neither pediatricians nor parents should put up with this.

SEVEN

Advocating for Children

Following my old heroes, I have always been an advocate for families and children. Ben Spock stood for families' rights and believed in their ability to raise their children wisely. D. W. Winnicott advocated for the support of parents in England. Their writings for and about families were a combination of psychiatry and pediatrics. I learned from both of them to value the insights and intrinsic ability of parents to nurture their own children. In my scholarly writing and hospital rounds, as well as in my popular books and television shows, I've tried to demonstrate that parents are the best experts. As I described in the previous chapter, the Touchpoints Program at sites around the country encourages care-givers to avoid a judgmental attitude and to recognize the passions and caring of parents. So many parents lack genuine support as they work to provide their children with optimal chances for their future. Such support depends upon relationships—relationships with medical professionals, with day-care providers, and teachers, as well as community resources. In today's economic and political climate, such support is not guaranteed, and we need to join parents in advocating to fund the programs they need.

Books for Parents

When I first began to write, I wanted to explain the marked individual differences that babies brought to their parents and how they might affect their relationship. Stella Chess and Alexander Thomas explored this in their work on temperament. Bill Carey, a colleague in Philadelphia, later adopted their concepts—especially the notion of a spectrum from active to quiet children—and applied it to pediatrics. My own experience with our very sensitive first child, Kitty, drew me to investigate these differences. Experience with the NBAS made me want to free parents from blame when the fit between them and their child was not an easy one. A quiet, sensitive child might be as difficult for an active, impatient parent as an active, impatient child for a quiet, sensitive parent. In 1968, I wrote an article about such a mismatch that might occur between parents and baby and how it might lead to failure in their attachment to each other. I submitted my article to Peter Davison at the Atlantic Monthly Press, who returned it, saying that it sounded like medical gobbledygook and that no one but a physician would ever read it. I was discouraged. But I turned to Peggy Yntema, also at the press, who suggested that I give it to Merloyd Lawrence. Merloyd and her husband, Sam Lawrence, had a firm copublishing with Delacorte Press. Merloyd encouraged me to use my ability to observe and describe behavior rather than to offer parents advice. She believed I had a "voice" that parents would listen to. I worked for nearly a year to write *Infants and Mothers*—a book about three children: (1) a very active child (Daniel), (2) a very quiet, sensitive child who was shy and withdrawn (Laura), and (3) an intermediate child (Louis). The book was based on the idea that, right from the first, a baby's temperament shapes his parents' reaction to him. If they were to make it with each other, the parents must consider how their approaches fit the baby's ability to take in, use, and respond to signals from the world. I learned this from Kitty, who, as a newborn, would close her eyes, shudder, and turn her head away from me if I rushed up to her and tried to reach her by touching, talking, cooing, and bouncing. I found I needed to use only one modality at a time—looking *or* touching *or* quietly talking *or* rocking—but I couldn't start with more or she'd shut me out. I had to respect her hypersensitivity if I were to reach and communicate with her. I learned so much from Kitty—as did a whole generation of parents!

Infants and Mothers, which first appeared in 1969, has sold over a million copies, and fifty years later I still receive thank-you notes from parents who have successfully "learned" to observe and trust their baby's reactions to their bids for interaction. The month-by-month chapters covered all aspects of each baby's development in the first year and the parent's adjustment to them as they grew together. I was often asked whether I was influenced by Spock or Winnicott. I digested both their approaches and wrote with their ideas intermingled with my own. Spock's *Baby and Child Care* gave parents permission to think of themselves and of their babies as individuals. Parents could learn how to respond by observing their baby and by being aware of how they had been cared for. Their own parenting was the basic experience from which they drew in learning their new roles. Winnicott, who was a famed psychoanalyst as well as a pediatrician, also emphasized both the natural wisdom of mothers and the childhood experience of parents, which Selma Fraiberg later named the "ghosts in the nursery." While drawing from these ideas, I based my writing on my own observations and the rich insights that working with parents gave me.

Infants and Mothers was so successful that Merloyd and Delacorte Press urged me to write other books. I was on my way. As I wrote, Chrissy would read and correct my writing at night. She was a great critic and often skeptical. She didn't really think I was a writer. One day the *New York Times* called and said that *Infants and Mothers* was brilliantly written. I said, "Can you hold a minute?" I called Chrissy to listen. "Now, can you repeat that?" Merloyd Lawrence stuck with me as editor through all my books. I always say that she put my medical writing into English. Without her, Peter Davison's ominous criticism would have come true.

After these publications, a publisher from Princeton came to see me. He offered me $5000 for the right to use all of my ideas in his own picture book for parents. It was a huge success, and he probably earned a great deal. I was naïve and not used to success. However, the money allowed Ed Tronick, Barbara Koslowski, and me to go to Africa and study the behavior of Zambian newborns.

Toddlers and Parents tried to rectify the fact that *Infants and Mothers* had been written for mothers. *Parents* included fathers too. *Toddlers* was one of the first books about two-year-olds and also became quite popular. *Infants and Mothers* was eventually translated into two dozen different languages and sold extremely well in Europe and Asia. *Toddlers and Parents* followed closely and has been translated in most of these countries, as have many of my books. The trilogy was rounded out by *On Becoming a Family*, which drew on Helene Deutsch's ideas about parents' preparation in pregnancy.

Doctor and Child was an attempt to ease the strain of a child's visits to the doctor. I was trying to empower parents to ask questions on each visit. The questions I mentioned earlier, "How am I doing as a parent?" and "Is my child developing well?" underlie all other questions that parents might bring and include emotional and behavioral issues as well as the usual worries about colds, stomachaches, and shots. I wanted to encourage parents to become their child's advocate. *Doctor and Child* set out to prepare parents, and, through them, the child, for what they would experience in the visit to the doctor.

Victor Vaughan, professor of pediatrics at Children's Hospital of Philadelphia asked me to edit two books for professionals with him: *The Family, Can It Be Saved?* and *The Family: Setting Priorities.* This gave me credibility in pediatrics groups around the country. Vic was an easy person to work with. These books were so successful that Barry Lester and I ran a roundtable for Johnson & Johnson in 1983 that was published as *New Approaches to Developmental Screening of Infants* (1983). During this time, my NBAS was beginning to be utilized and was the centerpiece for this work.

By 1984, Merloyd Lawrence had switched her imprint to Addison Wesley, and I went with her. Our first book there, *To Listen to a Child* in 1984 was an exhortation to pay attention to the infant's and child's behavior as their language. My goal was to help parents understand deviations and resistances at each stage of development in important areas like sleep, feeding, and toilet training and was aimed at avoiding conflicts by understanding the child's developmental issues.

In 1985, I responded to my daughters' advice: "Dad, our country has changed. Come out of the last century. Over half of women in this country must work outside the home today and they need your support. Write a book for working parents." *Working and Caring* was one of my most popular and influential books. Our country was (and still is) prejudiced about women who must leave their children in child care in order to work. I had been to France, where women had needed to work since World War II. The country not only developed good day care, the so-called *crèches*, as a major support for these working families but the culture accepted it and respected working mothers. Their subsidized child-care system with highly trained staff is a model from which we could learn. Having to leave small children in the care of untrained people whom they don't always trust is terribly painful to parents. In my book, I tried to explain the defenses parents set up against this grief, as I described earlier.

When good child care is not available, parent-infant attachment is bound to pay a terrible price. Ellen Galinsky at Families and Work Institute became interested in my work, and this institute has investigated what happens when working women and men are not provided with good child care or supportive policies at work in regard to their role as parents They have also advocated for family-friendly policies.

Published in 1992, *Touchpoints* sold nearly a million copies worldwide in its two editions. In *Touchpoints* I attempted to demonstrate for parents why regressions before a surge in a new development—cognitive, motor, and emotional—are necessary. I showed parents not to see such regressions as failures but as part of normal development. Readers were grateful to have these normal hurdles predicted, because they could avoid a cycle of worry and guilt.

In 2000, the distinguished child psychiatrist Stanley Greenspan and I published a book together, *The Irreducible Needs of Children*. The book was designed as a dialogue between a psychiatrist and a pediatrician outlining what we felt were the essentials to provide optimal environments for developing children today. This has become a textbook for institutions trying to back up young families. As we worked on it together, we found we disagreed a great deal. As we had to come to agreement if the book were ever to be published, we each learned a great deal. It was a great lesson in seeing how we can often learn more from disagreements than from too easy agreements.

Joshua Sparrow became a colleague and friend in 1991. As a child psychiatrist he brings a new generation's ideas and a brilliant mind to my clinical observations. Together we revised *Touchpoints* in 2006 and wrote *Touchpoints: Three to Six*, which was published in 2001 after several years of work. His wife is French and they were in Aix-en-Provence for a year for Wellesley College, where she teaches, so I had the happy necessity to travel back and forth to France, to work with him on the *Three to Six* book. Dr. Sparrow is a pleasure to work with as a coauthor. He also began to help me write my weekly column for the New York Times Syndicate.

With the hectic lives of parents today in mind, Josh and I have written seven small books on issues all parents must face, *Calming Your Fussy Baby, Discipline, Sleep, Feeding Your Child, Toilet Training, Understanding Sibling Rivalry,* and *Mastering Anger and Aggression.* The books, known as the Brazelton Way series, are pocket sized and can be read in a sitting. They are written for busy parents who might not have time to read a long book but would look at a short one that addresses their current burning issues. We hope these books reach an even wider audience and serve a preventive purpose. They also have been translated into many languages.

Launched in Paris

In 1982 Editions Stock in Paris licensed *Infants and Mothers* and translated it. It has been an important book for new parents in

France. Laurence Pernoud, my editor there, was the French guru for young parents. Every year, she published a very popular treatise for parents that her associates continue to update. Every parent there recognizes her work. Stylish and generous, she launched me in France—sharing her reputation and going on to publish most of my books there until she retired. We remained devoted friends until her death.

Because of the NBAS, a young filmmaker followed me with a newborn and made a documentary for a TV show in Paris entitled *Le bébé est une personne*. It was made in 1984 and has been shown on French TV for many years. The fact that the infant at birth could see, hear, and express himself and was even a competent little person was a new and very exciting idea there at the time. Claudine Amiel Tison, a neonatologist who had developed a neurological exam for babies, was very excited about my findings. She even took several kinds of behavior that were identified in the NBAS and added them to her own exam. She gave me a poster showing an active baby saying, "il est competent, competent, competent."

In addition to the TV film, Laurence's support and Dr. Amiel Tison's use of my concepts, a particular event made me known in France. The famous child psychoanalysts Serge Lebovici and Michel Soulé asked me to give the Princess Bonaparte lecture for the psychoanalytic society. Marie Bonaparte was a psychoanalyst, benefactor of the psychoanalytic movement, and member of the minor nobility. Serge was a force, influential in analytic circles around Europe.

Just as I was walking on stage to give the Bonaparte lecture, Dr. Lebovici took me aside and said, "You are the first American we've ever asked to give this lecture. There are over a thousand people in the audience (the largest crowd ever). I have three requests to you: (1) don't use your hands when you speak, (2) don't try to be funny, and (3) don't ever say anything you're not sure of." He was deadly serious. I looked him right in the eye. "Dr. Lebovici, you are asking me to give up the three things that every Frenchman does whenever he lectures." I stalked off and walked on to give the lecture. I did use my hands, I talked about newborns. I showed films and amusing pictures of small babies, and talked about my ideas about attachment. I discussed what the newborn baby brings to the equation to match the prenatal work of parents getting ready for the baby. I offered plenty of speculation. The major theme of my talk was to point out the many-sided competencies of the baby. The research I described from the NBAS, showing this, was entirely new. The audience seemed captivated and gave me a standing ovation. Everyone crowded around and I felt heady. Lebovici was obviously thrilled and relieved that I hadn't embarrassed him. (I wonder what he expected.) He said, "I want all of this fascinating work for us in France." Serge tapped Bertrand Cramer, a psychoanalyst from Geneva, "Bertrand, you go to America and learn all about this from Brazelton."

Bert came to Boston and we started a book together. It became *The Earliest Relationship*. It had a long gestation, five years, but was very successful in France and Switzerland and continues to sell well in the United States. It describes the stages of early attachment. Bert's contribution to *The Earliest Relationship* was his psychoanalytic case studies. Our book gives parents and professionals insight into the work and the dynamics of pregnancy and the early months. Bert and I drifted apart after a mischievous remark I made when we were on a panel together in northern France, and he described a case that he had given many times. When I was asked to comment, I said, "It seems interesting to me that all psychoanalysts steer their cases into events from their own past, so the child's issues are solved the way the analyst might have solved his own issues." Bert was not pleased.

I never hit the high again that I hit on that visit to Paris, although I have been there many times since. I was invited once to the Assemblée Nationale, where they were discussing how to upgrade their already advanced national child care. Arnold Sameroff, Joy Osofsky, and I were invited to the Assemblée to give our ideas about how to improve child care. *Working and Caring* had been translated into *A ce soir* (See you this evening). On the cover was a poignant three-year-old waving sadly at her mother who was leaving for work. Before our speeches, I was seated next to the wife of the president of the Assemblée. I said, "It is interesting you want our ideas from the US when your child care is so far ahead of ours." She responded gently, "That's what we want to hear. Please say that tomorrow." When I did the response in the press was enthusiastic.

More recently a Brazelton site for training in the NBAS was established in Paris. Drina Candilis is the director. An influential psychoanalyst, teacher, and therapist trained with the NBAS, she has brought attention to our work in France. There are also such Brazelton centers in Marseille, Geneva, Brussels, and in the United Kingdom at Cambridge.

Meanwhile, the spread of our research and the translation of my books led to other appearances in France. Hubert Montagner, a distinguished infant researcher asked me to come to the beautiful old city of Besançon to lecture about babies. It was an honor and a pleasure to meet him. He has made a particular study of infant behavior in child care. In a film he made of two seven-month-old boys in infant seats, sitting near each other, the infants smile at each other and even reach out for each other with their feet. As they do so, they moan quietly as if comforted. Then, if one of them is taken away from the other, he starts to cry. The one who is left hears him and joins in the crying. At another time, if his friend across the room and out of sight starts to cry, he hears it and becomes agitated. Infant researchers believe that this is evidence that babies are able to make significant relationships as early as seven months of age. This work has shown that babies in child care can learn whole new behaviors and suggests that they can form a relationship in addition to the one with their mothers and fathers as early as the second half of the first year. When adequately nurtured by a grandparent or a caregiver or paired with another infant, the baby demonstrates responses that say, "I know and care about you." The awareness of this can be threatening for working parents who wonder whether their baby will remain attached to them when left in substitute care. "Will he remember me?" "Who is most important to him?"

Reaching Parents Through Magazines

Baby Talk got me started writing for magazines back in 1968. It was run by a powerful warmhearted woman named Deirdre Carr. Having read my first writing on sucking, crying, and toilet training, she asked me to write for her magazine, given out free to new parents. DeeDee (as I came to know her) wanted me to write a page for each month of the baby's first year, and she would pay me one hundred dollars a page. Being paid for writing seemed like a dream. I took it on. I described a baby's behavior at each month and showed how his behavior helped us see inside his mind. The concept that a baby's behavior is indeed his language motivated my observations and became a theme in my writing.

Later, in 1972, *Redbook* magazine offered me a monthly column. Seymour Chassler (Sey) was a tall, distinguished man with a mustache, a quirky smile, and a very direct way of speaking. He would say, "We want *this* from you. Not what you've written. Now do it!" I felt comfortable knowing just what he wanted. He gave me a lovely editor, Kitty Ball Ross, to work with. Her husband, John Ross, a well-known psychoanalyst, was interested in fathers. Kitty and I would chat and giggle over each article. She'd give me her very sophisticated ideas. I'd tell her mine, and she'd tell me how she saw the article developing. The articles were picked up in France, Italy, and Spain and soon had the biggest readership in the magazine. Meanwhile, Ben Spock, Margaret Mead, and Jane Goodall were also writing for *Redbook*. It was becoming a thinking-woman's magazine, with a devoted audience of parents.

Redbook treated its writers to wonderful trips. On one, Chrissy and I, Ben and his first wife, and Margaret Mead were all sent to Puerto Rico, "in order to get to know each other." Ben was a fascinating man to talk to—psychoanalytically trained and with a very bright, inquisitive mind. We had a great time and became fast friends, comparing notes and ideas. He told me how much he'd enjoyed teaching at Case Western Reserve in Cleveland, how nostalgic he was after leaving the field. His life was now made up of public appearances and glitz. He was writing another book, trying to find a young pediatrician who would help him revise *Baby and Child Care*, which had sold many millions of copies—up there with the Bible. His success delighted him but also overwhelmed him. It made him re-evaluate his future, and he began to play a political role. He protested the Vietnam War, ran for president, and became an advocate for preservation of wildlands and natural resources.

In Puerto Rico, the four of us swam, ate, and drank together. We took a car and drove around the island. One day we drove up to the top of a mountain. Up, up, up, winding—winding forever. No people, no anything but trees. Finally, we found a little inn with a swimming pool. And it was hot, hot, hot. We'd been sweating in our open car. We were delighted to find civilization again. But the inn had a sign saying, "No one can use this pool but our overnight guests." Our hopes were dashed.

The owner, a plump Italian, came out to see our car. After we spoke, he recognized Ben. "Dr. Spock! Our hero! You helped us raise all thirteen of our children. My wife will be in heaven. Of course you can use our pool! We are so honored to have you here!" I realized the perks of being famous.

It was on that trip that I had a chance to pick Ben's brain about how he told girl babies from boy babies (clothed) from birth. He had been famous for this in Cleveland. Everyone admired his re-markable ability to observe. He was 80 percent accurate in distin-guishing the sexes, while no one else could get above 50 percent. "Newborn boys," he said, "are likely to have straight hair, little girls curly hair. Boys have V-shaped faces like their buttocks. Girls have round, soft faces." "Little girls look at you like this," and he made a gentle, heavy-lidded expression . . . "and little boys like this," and he made a wide-eyed, excited expression "as though expecting to be played with." This fit with my concept that the baby sets the tone for letting you know what he needs in the way of interaction with a caregiver.

When Ben divorced Jane years later and married Mary Morgan from Arkansas, he brought her to meet us in Cambridge. "Mary Morgan," as she was known, was thirty-four years younger and ran a child-care center where Ben had gone to lecture. After Ben's death, when Mary Morgan needed someone to help her revise his book, she called me and I referred her to Steven Parker at the Boston City Hospital. He helped her revise it once but after that experience was not willing to do it again. The commercialization of Ben's work is embarrassing for all of us in pediatrics.

Ben's son Michael ran the Boston Children's Museum, and through him I had an unusual opportunity. His wife, Judy, an artist, and I designed a great big toilet for the museum, big enough even for nine- and ten-year-olds to climb in and through to find out where their BMs had been going all these years. Children lined up for blocks to go through that toilet. No display ever quite caught children's interest as much. It showed me how much children feel they give up to become toilet trained. We expect them to feel urine or a BM coming on, hold onto it, go where we tell them to go, do it, and then watch it disappear. Children give away part of themselves to be trained.

Redbook dreamed up perhaps my most challenging assignment: I was sent to visit the Anderson quintuplets in Portland, Oregon. They were five healthy toddlers, and I was to write a series for *Redbook* on multiples. The Dionne quintuplets in Canada were the first-known surviving quints, but several of them had health problems. I was to spend a week with the Anderson quints, getting to know them and their parents. On the long airplane ride to Portland, I wondered what was wrong with me. Imagine agreeing to spend a week with five two-year-olds. I anticipated an ordeal.

Karen Anderson, the mother, was a remarkable lady. She already had two adopted children after six miscarriages. These older boys, four and three, had special needs and were in early intervention. She and Eric, the father, had almost given up on having their own. Then she became pregnant with five babies who survived and were normal and healthy.

Karen was delighted to have me visit her and to get to know her family. Eric, a burly salesman, was lovely with the children. He helped out a great deal, changing them, feeding them, cuddling them, playing ball with them. Karen was remarkably in control. For example, she changed the kids on the washing machine so she could just drop the dirty diapers in. She fed the five children at a specially designed circular table, with her in the middle, doling out bits of food to each one. She had a huge canvas under this table, which she hosed off afterward. She had it all figured out, and the five knew it.

Karen told me about her difficult pregnancy: toward the end of the fifth month, she could hardly breathe. It was a great relief when she went into labor at six months. But when the babies began to come, they were tiny preemies, all around one pound. The X-rays had predicted quadruplets, but after the fourth baby, a boy, appeared, the doctors realized that Karen's uterus hadn't emptied itself. Diane, the smallest and most fragile came last. She didn't breathe at first, so when she finally began to breathe, everyone in the delivery room let out a loud cheer. Karen says she'll never forget that cheer! The tiny fragile babies were frightening to behold and were immediately put on oxygen and IV lines for feedings and fluids, with nurses sitting around their bassinets. Everyone predicted ominous outcomes. "Will they survive? Do we want them to? If they do, the chances are over 50 percent that they'll be brain damaged." No one could promise the parents anything, even whether the babies would live. If they do, then the doctors said, "We'll see." There were so many hurdles to be gotten over.

This didn't daunt the Andersons. They both decided that the five were beautiful—three boys and two girls. They weren't. Premature babies at that stage are hairless; their heads are too large for the rest of their bodies. They have big eyes, scrunched up expressions, jerky movements interspersed with no apparent activity. Their faces are covered with tape to hold the oxygen tube in place; their scalps are full of tape to hold the fluid lines. Babies this size not only look fragile and frightening, they look like picked chickens. Only a parent could love them.

Karen did. She said she was determined they'd live and she would infuse them with life. In those days, parents were not welcomed into the ICU, and for the first day she complied. Then, she told me, she asked her husband to get her moved into a room near where they were being oxygenated and monitored. Each of the five monitors was clicking away. From her bed, she could hear all five monitors. She claimed that she first got to know her babies via their monitors. She prayed constantly for their survival. She never cried, never grieved. She just was determined that they'd survive and they'd be normal. When we talked later, her husband would nod and say, "She did it!"

When Karen finally was allowed to visit her babies, she claimed she already knew which ones were boys and which ones were girls by their monitors. Now, she wanted to know what to name them, so she studied them through the incubator walls. As she watched one baby, he threw off a vigorous fencing reflex, a tonic neck reflex. She named him Owen for a famous car driver. One girl seemed so demure and inactive. But she had a slight smile on her face. She named her Audrey for Audrey Hepburn. Each baby got a name that seemed to match his or her behavior in the incubator. "Then,

I knew they'd live. The next thing I had to face was whether they'd be OK. By the third day, I knew they would. And they are!"

Indeed, they were. At two, they were wonderful kids, active, responsive, friendly. When Karen asked them to say "hello" to me, they all stuck out their hands and looked me in the eye. Remarkable for a bunch of toddlers!

I began to see things I'd never seen before. In certain ways these five children were no more demanding than one or two might be. This was because they relied so much on each other. They were a team. When Karen wanted to change their diapers, they lined up at the washing machine. They already seemed to have recognized that she needed help, and they wanted to give it. I was amazed.

One story seemed to tell the tale. Roger, Owen, Audrey, Scott, and Diane were discharged after several months in the hospital. But Diane, the last born, was diagnosed with a cardiac lesion that needed surgery as soon as she'd reached ten pounds. At seven months, she was ready to be sent back to the hospital. All five had been sleeping together in one crib. When she was taken away, they all began to fuss, to cry out at night, to stop eating. They were really mourning her loss. When she came home, intact after her operation, they'd not yet learned to crawl. But they all pushed themselves up to her, put a hand on her, babbling, welcoming her. At seven months (minus three for their prematurity), they'd realized that one of them was missing. When they were reunited, they began to eat and sleep well and to grow again. Later, they all deferred to Diane. Whenever they were rough with each other, they never included her in their rough and tumble as if they remembered how fragile she had been.

After about four days, I dared offer to take them out into the yard. The Anderson's house was out in the country. The large yard

was fenced. No traffic, no predators, no dangers. Still, I was terrified. "What if one of these kids ran off and left the others—what
would I do?" All of a sudden, Scotty ran off. I tried to figure: "Do I
go after him and leave the rest or what?"

The other four realized Scotty had left them. They called out
to him: "Scotty! Scotty!" As if he felt guilty about leaving them,
he picked up a stone and held it up as if that was what he went
for. They all crowded around to examine THE STONE and were
herded together again. They showed me how they could take care
of each other.

I also learned more about how to deal with temper tantrums
from them than I've ever learned before or after. Again it was
Scotty, who lay down in the yard to have a rip-roaring temper
tantrum. All four of the others came up to try to stop him. Diane
lay down beside him to pat his face, Owen held his arms down, and
Roger threw cold water on him. Then Audrey had the answer. She
led the others away as if to ignore him. Scotty looked surprised and
stopped his tantrum. He sat up as if to say, "Why don't you pay attention to me? This is important!" I've recommended it to frantic
mothers ever since. "If you're in a safe place and can do it, just
walk away. The tantrum will lose its force."

Multiples learn so much from each other. And they are so important to each other. When parents or teachers wonder about
when to separate them, I say, "When they are ready. Not when we
are. They'll tell you when. This probably won't be until the children are five or six when they want different friends and different
experiences, but it may be later. But they'll always be close." I think
adults may be jealous of the intense relationships multiples develop
and thus feel in a hurry to separate them. But when they're not
ready, we should learn to wait.

Years later, I saw these five as young adults. They were hand-some, sturdy, effective young people. Karen wrote a book about her experiences, *Full House*, about how strong, determined parents can make successes out of seven children. She has become an advocate for multiples.

Family Circle magazine came to me in 1984 to ask whether I would be willing to think about moving to them after *Redbook* changed hands. It had been taken over by a new owner who wanted to make it a more "girlie, sexy" magazine. This came as a big surprise to us all. *Redbook* had won prizes for its leadership in journalism. I had certainly learned a lot from Sey Chassler and Kitty Ball Ross, who were being let go. *Family Circle* was a new and different oppor-tunity: it had a huge circulation, over half of which comprised lower-middle-class and minority families. That appealed to me tremendously. The editor, Jackie Leo, was a mother who'd read all my work, and she made me an irresistible offer. Although my prac-tice and hospital experience had been with all classes and ethnici-ties, I knew my writings so far had appealed mostly to sophisticated, highly educated parents. I wanted to broaden my ability to speak to all families. Ben Spock and Penelope Leach, two gurus for parents, had been successful in speaking to middle-class working parents, but I felt that their messages were too top down ("This is what you should do"). I wanted to be able to appeal to more disadvantaged, hard-to-reach sectors of our society. I hoped that *Family Circle* would help me bridge that gap.

Family Circle was a wonderful environment to work in. Susan Ungaro and Ellen Stoianoff were my editors. Later, Susan joined my Brazelton Touchpoints Center board and even led us as president of the board for two years. Ellen Stoianoff had been a magazine writer for many years and was to edit my articles for two decades. Josh

Sparrow, who became my coauthor in later years, says, "She made gold from hay." We would discuss the issue in some detail, the pros and cons, what might appeal to our audiences. Ellen suffered from rheumatoid arthritis, which seemed to make her even more sensitive and thoughtful. She understood my ideas and helped shorten and shape them to reach across classes and cultures. She criticized me, made me rewrite, condense, and become more punchy in my approach.

This great opportunity lasted until 2004, when Gruner and Jahr, the publishers, sold the magazine for reasons hard to fathom. The publication had been given every kind of accolade, and Susan had been given the highest magazine award for her efforts to reach out. Sales had grown.

My magazine days came to an end. However, my chance to write for a wide audience of parents had been expanded by my New York Times Syndicate column, which excerpted my books and also ran original pieces. Seventy to one hundred newspapers around the country subscribed. Josh Sparrow joined me later in writing the columns. Devoted readers show up whenever we lecture around the country. These wonderful magazines and our newspaper articles have given us the chance to be parent advocates and to press parents to advocate for themselves.

What Every Baby Knows

During these years, my advocacy for parents brought invitations to appear on talk shows, including from Oprah Winfrey. These brought both rewards and surprises. Barbara Walters spent a day with me taping our dialogue about what it meant to work outside the home. Then, she dropped the whole tape and used my ideas as her own.

I've been careful about such interviews ever since. On one of many tours for my books, a TV radio interviewer announced as soon as we went on the air that she had not read my book. We had an hour to fill. Taken aback, I said, "Well, it's not worth it to me or to your audience if you haven't done your homework." I got up and walked out of the studio. She gasped and took off her shoe to throw it at me as I walked away, leaving her to fill the hour by herself.

In 1982 I was offered my own TV show. Peggy Lamont, an agent, introduced me to three members of Tomorrow Entertainment: Hank O'Karma, Louis Gorfein, and Chuck Bangert. We called the show *What Every Baby Knows*, and it became a great success. We made new shows each year for thirteen years, from 1983 to 1996, and these continued to air afterward and in many countries around the world. We had a regular film crew, led by Bill Charette, that went with us for most of these years, along with a soundman, a helper, and Hank. I received an Emmy for my work. I learned so much from working with Hank O'Karma and his team. Our format was to find families with issues they wanted to share with other families; for this we traveled around the country. I was the discussant. We also showed children of different ages, observing and commenting on their behavior.

Many episodes stand out in our thirteen years of work. In one episode set in Marlin, Texas, a mother was teaching her three-year-old boy how to tell when one of newborn twin goats (kids) was sucking on the mother's teat. Goats always produce twins. The mother had once rejected a twin from an earlier litter, and it was important that this twin be accepted. One twin was already sucking successfully. The little boy's mother asked him to carry the newborn kid to her mother. It was already as big as he was, so he struggled to get it on the teat. When the kid had her mother's teat in her mouth and was apparently sucking, he said, "Mommy, I've done it!" His mother replied, "Not yet. Do you remember how to tell when she's really sucking?" The newborn kid's tail finally started wagging as she sucked successfully. He said, "Now I've done it!" The baby could suck nonnutritively, but until her tail started wagging, she was not really on the teat successfully receiving milk. This three-year-old learned the sign of successful sucking. His face beamed with success!

On another occasion, we were filming a newborn with his father, Jason, and his mother, Sally. I wanted to show them that he could imitate me and also that he knew his father's voice. I demonstrated to them that if I held him semiupright and alert in my hands and stuck out my tongue, he imitated me by sticking out his own tongue. I could even get him to imitate me with two tongue thrusts. Sally and Jason were ecstatic. To demonstrate that he would turn to a parent's voice, I held him in my hands, one hand under his head, the other one under his buttocks. When I spoke to him, he'd turn slowly to my voice. When Sally competed with me by speaking from his other side, he turned to her. She was amazed. She reached out to stroke him and said, "You know me already." Next, I asked Jason to compete with me by standing on the other side of me. Because only 80 percent of babies turn to their fathers, if he didn't, I was ready to tip his head toward Jason. But that was not necessary, and, when he did, Jason beamed. This show was one of our best.

Once we filmed a family named Jackson in which the mother and father were both blind. Their two-year-old, Johnny, was walking with his father down the street. Mr. Jackson and Johnny came to a curbstone. Johnny pulled on his father's arm to stop him. We'll never forget Mr. Jackson's delight. At just two, the child was already his father's helper. Not only was Johnny aware of his father's limitations, but he knew his father needed him to know when to stop at the curbstone to keep him safe from cars.

The thirteen years were productive, and people still remember the shows. I am often greeted by parents who watched them. Once, a flight attendant recognized me as I was sitting in the back of the plane. She asked whether I wasn't "the" Dr. Brazelton. She'd watched my shows and was grateful. "Do you want to sit in first class? Come on up. What would you like to drink?" "A martini." She brought me a big glassful (like a tub) and sat down next to me. "Now let's talk about toilet training," which I had to do all the way back to Boston for two and a half hours.

We went all over the continental United States and into Alaska filming our shows. Parents enjoyed the chance to share ideas and questions. They particularly liked the segments of each show in which they could recognize their own children's behaviors and development. Had we been funded for more shows, I would have been ready. I miss them. The ones we were able to complete and to broadcast have certainly been a chance for me to advocate widely for families.

Roadshows

In 1981, to spread the message of our research, we began the National Seminar Series, traveling from place to place, lecturing on our zero to three insights and assembling experts to join us. We have continued these, which we call our roadshows, for about twenty years. The fees we charge help pay for the Touchpoints Center. The first night, I talk to anywhere from one hundred to fifteen hundred parents. Most parents have the same questions. A sense of community arises as I refer parents to each other. The next day, three of my colleagues join me for a professional seminar day, usually speaking with 350–600 professionals. These pediatricians, nurses, child psychologists, and child-care personnel find they haven't really talked to each other even though they are doing the same work in parallel. They begin to feel a sense of community too and back each other up. We've done eight to ten roadshows a year all over the United States and have been asked to many cities several times.

We liked to think that we could construct a profile of each city from the questions that are asked. One night in Salt Lake City, Utah, the first respondent of the Q and A was a lady who stood up to say, "I was molested by my father. My mother was molested by her father. Now, I have a sixteen-month-old daughter and every time my husband goes near her, I wince. What should I do?" My immediate response was to advise her to get therapy quickly. "In that way, you can break the cycle. It's not fair to your husband or to your child to perpetuate that ghost from your own nursery—and you will if you don't get help." She was weeping, "That's what I want, but I don't know where to get it." I turned to the audience. "This mother has spoken bravely. Some of you now must go to her and tell her where to get help." No one moved. I said angrily, "This is the sickest city I've ever been in. Does no one want to help her?" At that point, two women got up and went to the microphone. "You're right! Salt Lake City is a sick, sick city. No one wants to help women here. If a woman has a problem she wants to report, it's quickly swept under the rug. Many of us have been molested in this polygamous society by our fathers and brothers but no one dares to report it and get help."

Whether this woman received the help she needed is unclear, but later we learned that women in Salt Lake City had begun to protest and things had started to change. Maybe we helped. Our roadshows often uncovered secrets that needed to be exposed. Many cities revealed their underbellies to us. That's what we were looking for, to stir up audiences to reach out to one another and pay more attention to family issues.

By the nineties we had banded together in a regular foursome who went on roadshows together—Kristie Brandt from Napa, California (a PhD nurse practitioner and expert on infant mental health), Maria Trozzi from Boston City Hospital (a grief expert), our own Joshua Sparrow (a child psychiatrist who speaks winningly on emotional learning and attachment, or on the touchpoints of adolescence), and me (I talk about the NBAS as an intervention and the first four months of attachment).

In 1996, we went to Tupelo, Mississippi, famous as the birthplace of Elvis Presley. Maria Trozzi and I were met in Memphis by two ladies with platinum, highly coiffed hair in a big Cadillac. They were to drive us to Tupelo for the talk to parents that night. On the way, as was our custom, we asked what the problems were in their town so we could address them or at least be aware of them as we talked. In their southern accents, the two ladies chirped, "Honey, we don't have any problems in Tupelo." "Oh, then why did you ask us to come down?" "Honey, we just wanted to meet you." "But don't you have any poor families, troubled children, or any drug problems?" "We surely don't know about any. You all just have a good time here." That night we talked to six hundred people in Tupelo and of course they had many, many problems.

We've visited nearly two hundred cities in the United States with our roadshows and seminars. In the past ten years, the focus has been on leaving each city with a hopeful program to back up the families who come together on the family night and the professionals who come together on the professional day. Before that, we'd get these cities and towns stirred up to be family friendly, but then we had to leave them with nothing to do about it. Now with our Touchpoint outreach project, we can offer a program for follow-up and support of stressed families. Community leaders gather at lunch to hear about our programs. At least fifty cities have followed up with Touchpoints training, setting up a site that can bring together family-centered health care, child care, and early intervention. Our roadshows have proven to be an entry into changing family support and policy in cities all over the United States.

On our travels, I always see old patients who come up to greet me or want me to sign one of my books. One night in Indianapolis, a woman with a fifty-year-old daughter crowded up to meet me. "I've always wanted Dorothy to meet you again. When we were studying at Harvard and penniless you used to care for Dorothy without our ever paying you. Now, we talk about you all the time. I remember one night when Dorothy was nine months old and had just learned to crawl. She crawled across the floor, found a penny, and swallowed it. I was frantic! I was about to call 911. But I called you first. After I told you she seemed happy and unperturbed, you said, 'Mrs. Johnson, why are you so upset about the penny? Do you need it? I can tell you how to retrieve it if you do. A penny can pass through with no problem.' I couldn't help but laugh and calmed down. We've never forgotten you as a result."

I loved my practice and have missed it ever since I retired in 1998.

Political Advocacy

In 1983, the March of Dimes (MOD) asked me to a dinner in Washington for an organization that they sponsored called Healthy

Mothers, Healthy Babies. I was to give the opening speech. Healthy Mothers, Healthy Babies was designed to be an outreach program for underserved parents and infants. The mission was to set up centers where young families could apply for supportive services. Meanwhile, the centers were designed to teach parents how to parent. The March of Dimes had invested in parent education as well as in early identification of children with special needs. Mary Hughes was the MOD administrator. George Miller, Pat Schroeder, Mary Jarrett, Christopher Dodd, cabinet secretaries, wives—many congressional and Senate leaders were to be there. I called Nancy Reagan's secretary to ask her whether she'd sponsor it and let me film her with a newborn. Her secretary said, "What a good idea. I'll ask her." (Anyone gets good press when filmed with a newborn baby.) I promised to arrange for a baby at the DC General Hospital. A week later, Mrs. Reagan's secretary called to say, "Mrs. Reagan can't go to the DC General for security reasons." "That's OK. I can bring the baby to her." "What a great idea. I'm sure she'll want to do it." Two weeks later, she called me and in ominous tones she said the visit was impossible. "Mrs. Reagan says she would rather talk about babies than hold them." I couldn't believe it, but it was the end of my association with Mrs. Reagan.

For the March of Dimes dinner, I instead made a film I've used ever since—one segment of a two-day-old newborn's competent behavior and a second segment of a two-month-old interacting with his mother and demonstrating the rhythms, the nonverbal rise and fall of attention-nonattention. This rhythm demonstrates the baby's need for homeostasis. The mother learns this from her baby very quickly. First, she alerts the infant. He responds by smiling, vocalizing. Then, he turns away and she lets up on him to recover. Then they interact again—until he is overwhelmed. This rhythm becomes the basis for early communication and for speech later. You speak. I speak. Meanwhile, this kind of communication is teaching a small baby how to be alert and responsive to an adult's exhortations, then recover and prepare for the next exchange.

The film also showed how, by two months, a baby would respond differently to a mother and a father. With the mother, everything about the baby is gentle, reaching out, coming back—fingers, toes, mouth, and eyes. Even heart rate is slow. The baby will respond to her for three to four responsive cycles, and by two months this becomes an expectancy in the baby—a cognitive expectation. With the father at two months, the baby responds differently. Fathers tend to sit back and poke a baby from bottom to top—three to four times per minute. So at eight weeks, the baby expects to be played with. Face and eyes light up, fingers, toes, heart rate are all sped up, motions are jerky, reaching for play. We also showed the "still face" film described in Chapter 3, in which the mother violates the interactive rhythm. Only after the mother begins responding again is the baby relieved.

When I showed the films to the large March of Dimes in DC (without Mrs. Reagan), they all stood up and cheered. It was a major launch for an organization that the March of Dimes thought might increase public awareness of the desperation that families in our country face. It gave me a presence in DC and in Congress, which I've used since. We sat at a table with George Miller, Pat and Jim Schroeder, Judy Woodruff (then an anchor at CNN) and her husband. Pat Schroeder's husband, Jim, was a Princetonian, so we had that in common. Pat allowed me to become part of her team. Later, she helped me with the bill for parental leave. She also took us around the south to alert governors and their congressional leaders to the need for more parental support. On the tour of the southern governors, we went to various mansions in North and South Carolina, Mississippi, Georgia, and Arkansas. The highlight was Arkansas. It was obvious that Bill Clinton had the making of a president: charm, charisma, and brilliance. Hillary was strong and determined as the state's first lady and a great advocate for families and children. I fell for her in Arkansas and followed her road to the White House. I was grateful for her support in our advocacy work. They both are stars, real leaders, and we have been friends ever since.

The MOD program Healthy Mothers, Healthy Babies, however, never really thrived. There are a few centers around the country but not as many as expected, despite the desperate need. Mary Hughes resigned at MOD, and my involvement went with her. Later, what we learned from our Touchpoints programs highlighted one of the defects: you don't "tell" parents how to parent. You support them, you give them advice when they ask for it, but you don't tell them what to do. They learn from their mistakes as well as from their successes. Learning to parent becomes a combination of reading the child's behavior and being aware of the experiences and biases from your own past (the ghosts from your own nursery). Being told how to parent can even be demoralizing if the instructor seems to be saying, "I know but you don't."

During these years Zero to Three: National Center for Infants, Toddlers, and Families, was a great support, offering me more research to add to my own and back up my advocacy. The late Emily Fenichel was the brain behind this and I am eternally indebted to her.

In 1986 I worked with George Miller in the House and Christopher Dodd in the Senate on a bill to expand services for children with special needs. Rep. Miller called me to Washington to testify before the Select Committee on Children, Youth and Families. As always when I testified, my testimony was followed by a perfect little family—mother, father, two children (boy and girl) all dressed up. After I beseeched the government to pay attention to families and invest in them, this family would testify: "If you follow Dr. Brazelton's advice and the government pays for such family supports, you will take away family choice." I wondered what choice they were claiming that most families had. Our country has continued to act as if all families, however needy, can manage their own affairs without any support. Our opposition claimed that the government should not be supportive, because each family "chose" to live the way they did. However, the bill passed, becoming Public Law 99–457, the Education for All Handicapped Children Act. To me, this was one of the most important bills that Congress has ever passed. Not only have we been able to fund programs all over the United States for families of children with special needs, but we have also learned so much—about the brains of these children, about how early intervention can help children with impairments to manage and even overcome them. All of this has since been confirmed by brain imaging techniques.

My testimony was also used by George Miller in the House and Chris Dodd in the Senate to fight for the Family and Medical Leave Act. John Kerry and Daniel Moynihan were powerfully important in supporting the bill. In spite of the testimony of those perfect middle-class families, the bill was passed in 1993.

On one of my trips to DC, I was asked to visit, to consult, and to lecture at Gallaudet College, a college for the deaf. Deafness in infancy is a huge challenge. Often, in those days, it was not diagnosed early because these babies appeared to have autism. They would rock back and forth, as if to fill up the silence. At Gallaudet, I was introduced to signing as a form of communication between parent and infant. It was necessary as a substitute for hearing in early parent-infant interaction when a baby is profoundly deaf. This early pattern of communication helps to diminish their isolation. Parents were taught to begin signing to their infants in the first few months. They were taught how to encourage the babies to sign back as early as the first year. The autistic behavior disappeared, and this gestural communication, back and forth, brought out unexpected results in these tiny infants. Their development was no longer delayed. Parents understood the experience of their deaf babies and what it might have meant to them to live without communication. This was one way in which our work on parent-infant interaction in the first few months was taking new forms.

Whenever I testified in the House or Senate about how critical it is to give new parents time to get to know their new babies and themselves as parents, senators and representatives seemed to see only the dollar signs of freeing up paid employees. No one expected to pay parents on leave, although Sweden had demonstrated that a year off was really productive for the economy and very important to young families. Because we had been successful in getting our parental leave passed, we thought it was time to set up a PAC: "Let's go for parents. We'll offer them the backup in DC they need to get action. All we need from them are their names and votes."

Bernice Weissbourd and I began to plan for an organization called Parent Action. We hired a wonderful woman from Baltimore, Rosalie Street, to run it. We did as much PR as we could afford. We thought parents would lap it up. On each of my roadshows, we'd have fifteen hundred families present. They'd all be enthusiastic, but only ten would sign up. After years of struggling to get backing, we had little success. Parents would say, "What a great idea but I just don't have any time or money to give to it." Although we offered to do the legwork, it seemed as if we just couldn't get enough energy or passion from parents to make it work. We finally had to give up

Several others have tried to do what we did. Rob Reiner, a Hollywood director deeply committed to families, tried to use movie stars to do this without much success. Parents today are too pressed by their own lives and may also feel hopeless about getting any support from government. Maybe they also do unconsciously worry about whether the government regulation might take away "choice."

The Clintons and Child Advocacy

When the Clintons got in the White House, Hillary was very much on our wavelength. Bettye Caldwell, the pioneer in early child development, had known and worked with her in Little Rock. Marian Wright Edelman, the CEO of the Children's Defense Fund, had been a good friend of Hillary's and was very much behind her.

After meeting her in Arkansas with Pat Schroeder, I got to know her better in the White House. She included me in her White House conferences to raise awareness of some of the issues facing parents and children. The conferences were on topics such as effects of poverty on children's development, early intervention for children with special needs, child care and its importance for working families, and research on brain development. There was also one on women's issues and their importance to families. These White House conferences consisted of audiences of one to two hundred specialists, ten to twelve speakers, and lots of publicity. Hillary did more for families and children than any other first lady. In the 1950s through the 1980s there had been a White House conference every ten years to alert the country to important issues about children and families. These had been discontinued when the Reagans took office. For those of us immersed in these issues, it was an exciting opportunity to have them revived and to share ideas with other clinicians and researchers.

For example, at the brain research meeting, Harry Chugani, a neurologist from Ann Arbor, showed films of newborn babies' brains. These showed how the brains lit up in certain small areas when objects were presented to the baby. When the mother leaned over to pick him up, the whole brain lit up. What an example of the importance of learning from interpersonal interaction!

My association with the Clintons gave me a huge boost in advocating for children. One day I was in Decatur, Illinois, with Claudia Quigg on her wonderful *Baby Talk* program when I had a call from the White House. Mrs. Clinton's aide said, "Dr. Brazelton, Mrs. Clinton would like you to be with her tonight when President Clinton announces the health care bill." "I can't possibly get there. I'm in southern Illinois." "She will be so sad. She wanted you and Dr. Koop to ride in the motorcade with her." At the thought of riding in the motorcade, I instantly agreed. "I'll get there. Don't worry!" I had no idea how I'd get from Decatur to Chicago to Washington, but I was determined to do it. It never occurred to me to ask for a presidential plane.

I made it back to DC and was on hand for the motorcade. Dr. Koop and I were treated as a package. He was the head of Health and Human Services and very much my superior and senior. It was absolutely wonderful to be picked up by the Secret Service and put in the back of a long, black limousine (which reminded me of my grandmother's car when I was little). Koop and I were ushered to our first-row balcony seats in this huge auditorium. The cabinet was right behind us. I was seated next to the wife of the Speaker of the House of Representatives. On my other side, between me and Koop, was a vacant seat. We kept wondering whom it was for. After a roll of drums, trumpets, and big fanfare, in came Hillary to sit between us. I was so excited and delighted that I hugged and kissed her—in front of the news cameras! I realized too late that men don't kiss the wife of the president in public. But she loved it—and I enjoyed every minute of her company.

When the president's speech came on for him to read, Hillary realized it was the wrong speech—the one from last week. She said, "Oh God: He won't know what to say about the health care bill." But he did. He gave a superb speech—off the cuff. As he began to speak powerfully, she began to relax. I leaned over to her and said, "Hillary, you want to have some fun?" "Yes," she said. So I said, "Let's measure the latency before the Republicans clap after each important point he makes." She was delighted. As the latency got longer and longer and as he became more and more eloquent, she began to gloat: "I think we are winning!" I wish she'd been right. We didn't get the universal health-care coverage at that time. Sixteen years later, Obama had the guts and the clout to get it passed.

Sitting in the midst of all those famous people, names I'd heard and read about, was a blast. I could watch their faces from my balcony seat. It was one of my fondest moments, but I was sad that none of my family or Boston friends were there.

John Kerry, Chris Dodd, Pat Schroeder, and George Miller all came up afterwards. Bill Clinton on the way out was shaking everyone's hand. When he came to me saying, "Hi Berry!" I said, "What a brilliant speech and an exciting presentation!" He retorted, "I hope I did as well as you do, Berry, on your television show!"

Hillary and Bill were great supporters of our work. Later, when she was in the Senate, I took Josh Sparrow to meet Hillary. She greeted us warmly and took us down to her office in the Senate building.

"Berry," she said, "I know how to help you in this administration. I'll just disagree with you and then they will turn toward you."

Bill once came into a crowded gymnasium in Harlem, when Geoffrey Canada was celebrating the opening of his new school. Across the crowded room he said loudly, "Berry Brazelton! What a great place to see you." What a memory, and what diplomacy! The Clintons' advocacy has been an important milestone in changing our country's attitude toward children and families. But we still have a long way to go.

EIGHT

Advocating for Families
Around the World

I n the 1970s and '80s I began to have opportunities to spread
my ideas about newborns and early intervention around the
world. My first chance came in 1977. The US Department of
Health, Education, and Welfare sent six pediatricians to Krakow,
Poland, to confer with others there about what could be done to re-
pair the lingering aftermath of the Nazi destruction of Poland thirty
years earlier. Bob Haggerty, Joel Alpert, and I were three of those
sent, as we were interested in family and child development. In this
magnificent old city, we conferred about preventive measures to
improve family life and ways to use our growing knowledge of child
development. In Warsaw, we saw the plight of teenagers raised by
a traumatized generation of parents, with problems of drugs, violence, and depression. We were able to recommend programs for
young parents, beginning at birth, to help them past the sense of
hopelessness transmitted by older generations. We recommended

early intervention and support for new parents from the first and continuing access to help whenever they reached an impasse with their children.

Caracas: An Intractable Cycle of Poverty

Another opportunity came in 1980 when I was asked to lecture in Caracas, Venezuela. Luis Machado, then in the newly designed position of minister of the Development of Human Intelligence, wanted to change education and the situation of families. Venezuela was a typical South American two-class society—very rich and very poor. As a result, violence and theft were a part of life in Caracas. The well-to-do lived in fenced-in enclaves guarded by vicious dogs, with broken glass atop the walls. Anyone who committed a minor infraction in the city was likely to be killed, not incarcerated. Children were starving and begging on the streets.

Machado saw that education could break the cycle of poverty. His talented assistant, Beatriz Manrique, had read my papers and books and set up speaking engagements for me in Caracas. Crowds of mostly well-to-do parents came to each lecture. Beatriz came to Boston to be a fellow in my child development program.

Beatriz and I began to develop educational programs. We conceived of starting with parents from the first, educating them so that they in turn would value education in their children. It didn't work as well as we had hoped, because survival had to be the primary goal. Without the assurance of programs for food and housing, education was just a frill. We became discouraged. Machado was eliminated from the government, and those at the top did not see that deep poverty could be improved by education combined with basic support. Yet we still believed that if you started from birth with families, you could have a powerful effect on the outcome of children. Later, Beatriz established TV programs for mothers on the delivery floors at the maternity hospitals in Caracas. They were extremely popular. There was great hunger for improvement of children's welfare in the face of the continuing plight of the underclass in Caracas. What a vision, and what a disappointment it was not to be able to carry out our programs there. But I hear that her efforts have continued and have had some success in improving the plight of lower-class families and their approach to education.

New Delhi: Schooling and Development

That same year, I was sent to New Delhi on a United States–India commission to consult on a particularly interesting problem. Six US and six Indian experts were sent to look into a study Indian researchers had designed. Whenever a new building was being constructed in the city, both mothers and fathers were hired to work on it. This meant either leaving the children with a friend or relative or having to bring all children in the family to take care of each other on the building site. Most families with more than one child chose the latter, relying on the older children to care for the younger ones. Instead of being in school, children of all ages were playing together, unsupervised, as the building went up. Since it took months or even years for each project, none of the children were receiving any kind of formal education.

Indian investigators were studying whether, if they offered schooling to these children right on these sites, it would make a significant difference in their development. These children came from the lowest castes of India, so they had a feeling of hopelessness about their potential. The parents felt this as well. They thought of their children as having a future similar to their own—working sixty hours a week in order to survive. The children, however, were eager for the instruction that the investigators provided. Most of them lapped it up. Their IQs had registered between 70 and 90 at the beginning of the study. The teaching was so successful that their scores rose twenty points on average—a brilliant outcome for any intervention. We advised the investigators to look also beyond cognitive gains to longer-term benefits such as finishing high school, staying out of trouble, ambition for getting jobs, contributing to society in some way or other, caring for their families, and rising out of poverty and into a less vulnerable lifestyle.

Our team all walked as a group around New Delhi. We felt overwhelmed by the noise, the colors, and the touching (everyone wanted to touch, to grab, to beg from us as tourists). There were many children with disabilities in the streets, some of whom turned out to have been mutilated by their families so as to make more successful beggars. One day, Bettye Caldwell made the mistake of giving some coins to one little child with a disability. As a result, we were constantly followed by swarms of children, all begging, "Please, Mister. Can't you see I'm crippled?" It was a frightening horde. Soon it became almost impossible for us to go sightseeing except protected by a bus. We realized the vast extent of poverty in India, and our dreams of doing anything about it were much diminished. However, the project for the families working in building sites held lessons for other projects in India.

South Africa: Two Audiences

Over the years, Johnson & Johnson made several opportunities to work for children abroad possible. In the United States, they have supported pediatric research: backing studies, convening experts, and then publishing the resulting monographs. This included one about our research with the NBAS and early intervention. Another, on early attachment, featured our face-to-face research.

Johnson & Johnson asked me to go to several countries around the world to lecture on infancy and parenting. Things were different in those days, and I was not expected to mention Johnson & Johnson products. I could spread the word about the work we had done with parents and infants, helping to improve the outcome for children in these countries. The support was vital to my research and to my mission. Johnson & Johnson also provided grants to make films of parent-infant development. They helped us set up a Brazelton Center for work with newborns in Boston and Chicago and eventually in a dozen cities around the world. These centers are all run by dedicated pediatricians who are training other professionals on my NBAS and on early infant-parent interaction. They have no ties to Johnson & Johnson.

In 1983, I visited South Africa. Apartheid was still in effect. Black men were often torn away from their families to be sent to work in other parts of the country with no promise of return. As a result, women were left with their children to support. Their only resource was often to take on housework for white middle-class families. As a result, children were often left alone for the day or in neighbors' homes or in orphanages. These orphanages, set up in each township (the slums where these desperate parents lived), were run by Catholic nuns. Mothers left their children there all week. On weekends, they'd come to gather up their children and spend the weekend on the grassy slopes around the orphanage.

We were asked to give lectures in the four biggest cities in South Africa: Johannesburg, Durban, Port Elizabeth, and Cape Town. The organizers in South Africa anticipated audiences of a thousand in each city, and to my surprise they turned out to be right. Fearing that the audiences would be all white, I asked to speak to black audiences as well. "All your audiences will be mixed, don't worry" (mixed meant Indian, then referred to as "colored," as well as white). I knew what mixed meant and insisted on including black people. "But we can't get black people into our audiences." "Then, I can't come." They were shocked. One month later they called to say that they'd arranged a black audience in each of the four townships adjacent to the cities so that I could lecture to whites and Asians in the places they'd originally arranged. I felt a sense of achievement.

Johannesburg was a sprawling city of more than 5 million (probably not all blacks were counted in that number). Desmond Tutu asked us to have an audience with him. He was terribly grateful for our stance in regard to black parents. Winnie Mandela (Nelson was in jail at the time) came to my lecture in Soweto. Soweto was a muddy, smelly collection of cardboard houses with tin roofs. Children were starved looking, with ribs stuck out, pop-eyed, and staring. They'd surround me, pushing to touch me or rob me or just to feel my clothes and my skin. I visited the orphanage there—children indoors, mostly asleep on their dirty cots—waiting for the weekend and their mothers' visits. Black nuns swished back and forth in the corridors, too overwhelmed with their jobs to give the children the loving attention we all knew they needed. We saw a few children in the muddy playground, playing with a ball made of tied string and a branch of a tree for a bat. Even the dogs were pitiful. They were scrawny, all bones and cowering stances. The rats seemed to be the best-fed and most vigorous, satisfied residents. The black leaders of Soweto tried so hard to show me the best of their township. No white person visited from Johannesburg; danger but also guilt kept them away.

In the townships we saw no men, only women, caring for the children. Any woman at home in these cardboard houses was surrounded by children. I noticed that the children I saw at home were more alert, more energetic than those in the orphanage. Just a mother's presence gave them courage and energy.

When I was given a chance to meet with about thirty-five black mothers, assembled in one mud brick building, I had no idea what to say to them. I'd never experienced so much poverty and desperation. My work had been with middle-class parents whose main question was whether to work or stay at home, not the stress of never having such a choice. I was anxious, and I'm sure I conveyed this to my passive, dutiful audience. As expected, each black mother in the audience had several children around her skirts. Seeing a baby in the front row, I asked the mother whether I could play with her—a tiny, old soul, about three weeks old, clinging to her mother's slack breast.

When we took her off the breast, she whimpered weakly but relaxed when I held her close to me. I cooed softly to her and rocked her gently. As I did, she began to come to an alert state, looking around. She looked up into my white face. I rattled my rattle softly in one ear and then the other. She turned each way to find it. When I used my red ball, she followed it almost hungrily. Now all the mothers were standing up and crowding in to see what I was doing. I got her to walk by using her walk reflex. Everyone murmured softly. As I held her and let her follow my face and my voice from one side to the other and up over her head, her own face was bright and alert. By now, the audience was fascinated. I talked softly to her; she leaned toward me and even tried to coo. Her mother came up to me. I thought she might want to take her baby back. Instead, she began to rub her arm against my arm. I said, "What are you doing?" Through a translator, she replied, "I want to rub your magic from your skin into mine!" The thirty-five ladies lined up to rub their arms against mine. "You are a magician. You make our baby sing!"

From then on, we were in communication with each other. Each mother brought me her child to "bless" and to "make him sing like that baby." I played with each one a bit. Despite the malnutrition, each child was so ready for any playful interaction that most of my efforts were successful. By that time, they all wanted to tell me of their plight, and they wanted to give their children what they could. I promised them that we would get toys and books that they could use with their children.

During the visit to the townships I realized that the "orphanages," overwhelmed though they were, were really child-care centers for these working women. They could leave their children there while they went off to work. When I had the chance with Desmond Tutu or other sympathetic leaders, black or white, I urged them to consider setting up training sites for young women to prepare them for taking care of and nurturing children in the child-care centers they needed.

It was difficult to tear away from these impressions of the townships and the poverty and hardship we saw in each of them and then to focus and relate to the middle-class white audiences. Yet, our audiences kept getting bigger and bigger. We had press and many leaders, including the Afrikaner president of South Africa, ask to talk to me about preventive care and what could be done.

The Language of Babies: Sydney to Hong Kong

In 1989 I went to Australia to lecture in Sydney, Melbourne, Brisbane and then on to Asia. The chief of pediatrics at Children's Hospital in Sydney, Kim Oates, had trained at Children's Hospital in

Boston. He had me give grand rounds to introduce me to the professionals in Sydney. Penny Alexander, a professor of psychology at the university, Beulah Warren, also a professor there, and Marianne Waugh, a physiotherapist, had come to Boston to be trained on the NBAS. They were now known in Sydney for this training. As a Harvard professor in pediatrics, I had certain credibility; our lectures were crowded each time. We were also urged to come to Melbourne to their prestigious Medical School and Children's Hospital. Another ex–Children's Hospital pediatrician, Frank Oberklaid, was a professor there.

We went out in the country to the famous Ayres Rock—four hours from Sydney and the coast. There, the Aborigines still lived, having been treated by the Aussies in the same way we've treated Native Americans in the United States. The "Abos" have been driven out of good farmland into the too dry or too wet interior. They have survived, but their culture is deteriorating. Many of the men we saw were alcoholic, the women weary, and the children not thriving, cultural throwaways. It was a depressing picture—such a contrast to the Texas-like prosperity of the farmlands around the thriving cities.

From Australia we went to Japan. By that time, I had been back and forth to Japan several times to study babies and children for our research on the Goto Islands off the western coast of Japan, as mentioned in Chapter 4. I had gotten to know many of the pediatricians in Japan through my friend Kobey, professor of pediatrics at the Children's Hospital in Tokyo. Johnson & Johnson arranged lectures for me in Osaka, Tokyo, and Nagasaki. They always seemed well attended, even though I knew I'd said the same things to many of the same people on previous visits. But the Japanese are so polite and graceful. They would nod all the way through my lectures. Now, I think they were nodding because I had said it before and they were becoming more and more familiar with my thinking. I talked about newborns, the wonderful, gentle, alert Asian babies we shared. I talked about the face-to-face paradigm through which we'd learned so much about the early attachment process between parents and babies. By then, I could also talk about our work on the Goto Islands. Most of our audience was not familiar with this wonderful part of their own world. We were learning a great deal from this study. Since then, research sites in several Japanese cities continue with training in the NBAS.

Singapore was the next stop. Away from the squalor, the overpopulation, and the poverty that affects so many Asian countries has arisen this gleaming, clean, disciplined, well-organized city. It was impressive. Crime was said to be almost nonexistent, perhaps because of strict enforcement of laws. While we were there, an American teenager was jailed for having written graffiti on the walls of a building. Poverty appeared to be at a minimum. There certainly were no homeless people or derelicts on the streets. At that time, as far as we could tell, there was no variability in the way people lived. No very rich and no very poor. Yet people seemed emotionally flat there: neither depressed nor very happy looking.

However, our ideas about newborns, attachment, and early intervention were lapped up. The medical school asked me to repeat my lectures so "everyone could hear them." The then president's daughter was a pediatrician, so she was eager to show us around. We had an enthusiastic though not very exciting reception. Although it was fascinating and enlightening to see how a government can optimize life for everyone, there seemed to be little passion for living left. To me, this suggested that changing a culture in a short time had a cost.

. In Thailand, we met with Nittaya Kotchabhakdi in the pediatric department of Ramathibodi Hospital, their largest. An MD, MPH, especially interested in child development, she had been in Boston and trained with me, so she was eager to entertain us. Her husband, Nick, a professor of neurology and neurological science, is from an old Thai family. She is Chinese, one of seven children. Her father and mother came from China to set up a little food store in downtown Bangkok. By hard work, they raised seven children, supporting the education of each all the way to doctorates. Bangkok was already a fairly modern city, rapidly becoming more so. The rich were rich, the poor very poor. Nittaya had performed a miracle, which UNICEF quotes to this day. She went by motorbike to all the little villages in Thailand, where she'd immediately ask for a meeting of elder women and young mothers. She'd get their confidence by playing with their babies. Then she'd address a tragic custom in Thailand. Mothers were discarding their colostrum, calling it dirty milk. Of course, their breast milk didn't come in until the third or fourth day, so new babies had nothing for the first few days. By that time, they were often too weak to stimulate their mother's breast milk. Breast feeding was becoming less successful. The formula the villages produced was often watered down and not adequate to the babies' needs. And it certainly didn't contain the antibodies necessary to combat infections. So, babies were dying unnecessarily.

After Nittaya played with their babies, showing the infant's potential from her demonstration of the baby's behavior (based on my NBAS) the villagers were ready to listen to her argument. "Don't throw away the colostrum—it will make better babies for you. And breast feeding will be more successful!" Breast feeding began to increase again, infant mortality declined, and awareness of this success spread. UNICEF used this experiment as a magical example of

what one person could do to change maladaptive customs in a developing country. Nittaya became a hero. She saw how newborns
can open the door to change in a culture.

Whenever we gave a session on parents and infants, and we gave
many around Bangkok and Thailand, the princess was there to introduce us. She rarely stayed to hear my lectures, but she made
clear her support for Nittaya and me. At one point, she asked for us
(Nittaya, Chrissy, and me) to come to the palace. I was thrilled: (1)
it was the palace of *The King and I*, (2) I'd never been received by
a princess in a palace before, and (3) I thought maybe it meant
she was really going to back Nittaya's work with royal funds, which
she was.

We were told we'd have a fifteen-minute session and to bring my
books as a present for her. We arrived on time and were ushered
into one of the gorgeous rooms at the palace. Our presents were
placed on golden trays to offer to the princess. When it was time for
our fifteen-minute interview, everyone in livery got down on hands
and knees. In Thailand, no one is ever supposed to be the same
height as royalty. The retainers, garbed in dazzling costumes, all
skittered across the floor. Even Nittaya kneeled and bowed down.
We didn't and we offered our hands to her to shake—in typical
American fashion. She was lovely and gracious, about forty-eight or
forty-nine, a little bit worried looking, or maybe just concerned. She
welcomed us warmly. We all sat around on gold chairs. The servants
fed us tea and delicious cakes as we started chatting politely.

By way of conversation, I said, "You seem to have to be at one
meeting after another as your duty to open and sanction them."
Nod. "It must seem pretty tedious." Nod. "Do you like your job?"
She looked at me in utter surprise. Her whole face then changed
into a smile. She answered, "No!" Our fifteen-minute interview

lasted over two hours as she told us how boring her job was. How she felt obligated to fill the shoes of her royal position, but how little real reward there was. She didn't actually express it, but one could see the resentment she suppressed over taking on such a lonely, responsible job while her rake of a brother shirked all responsibility. Her father, at that time king, had been born at Mount Auburn Hospital in Cambridge. She felt a kindred spirit in us from that link with Cambridge. In her two-hour confession, she let us know how she wished she could have been a practicing pediatrician taking care of babies and families. She said to me, "What gratification you must have." At the end of the interview, we felt so close to her, so sad for her. Afterwards, she promised Nittaya to back her in setting up a center for parents and children in Bangkok.

Everywhere I lectured in Thailand, there were hundreds of eager young faces. Although I spoke only in English, they had simultaneous translation and seemed to understand, nodding at the right time, laughing at my jokes. Nittaya had sent her best students to train as fellows with me, including Dr. Tom Sambakya, a brilliant young pediatrician who became her right-hand colleague. I've returned to Bangkok many times since, once to help Nittaya open her center. Saffron-clad monks chanted for hours at her opening— a first for our work around the world!

Outstanding in my memory of this trip through Asia is being taken to visit the largest orphanage in Seoul, South Korea. It had been a large source of adoptions for families in the States. These Korean babies were so impressive, intact neurologically, very gentle, and well organized. Their adoptive families were lucky. At the time of the Olympics, the Korean government tried to play down the reputation of South Korea as a major source of adoptable babies. This diminished the opportunities somewhat, but South Korea remains one of the countries from which international adoptions are most often arranged.

I wanted to see this orphanage, for I'd had several of these great babies in my practice. Because of these adoptions, I had learned to warn adoptive parents not to rush to hug, talk to, and look at the small baby who had just come into their lives. As the baby left the environment he had adjusted to and lost his previous caregiver, he was likely to be overly sensitive to any change. If parents (still strangers) rushed to hug him and bounce him, they would be stressing his whole system. If they talked too loud or too insistently—"Hello, baby. Welcome! Look at me!"—his auditory system would overload. If they looked him steadily in the face, it would overload his visual system. On the other hand, greeting him quietly and gently and waiting for him to respond would give him necessary time to adjust his hypersensitive systems and to be able to take in the new environment.

My experience with Asian babies, quiet motorically and sensitive auditorily and visually, made me feel that their rhythms as well as their sensory modalities were often overwhelmed in their new homes. Given time to adjust, they became more able to respond to a new caregiver. With the eager greetings of a new parent, the baby might withdraw and curl up into a shell, disappointing the yearning caregiver with what appeared to be a negative response. The attachment process could easily go off track. Given time however, the new baby would be ready, even hungry, for attachment to the adoptive parents. The necessity to grieve for the old environment and to adjust to the new could be expected to take one month if the baby was four to six months old, six weeks if six to twelve months, and even longer for an older child. Adoptive parents need to be warned to wait this out. This warning protects them from feeling disappointed and rejected by the baby's initial reticence.

At the orphanage, all the children who could walk rushed up to us. They held out their arms to be picked up, to be loved. If you picked one up, though, she would squirm to get down. Their experience with being loved was too thin. Too much overwhelmed them.

The children's eagerness to follow, to be picked up, to be hugged, however superficial, certainly had its effect on an adult. I found myself yearning to take one—or two or three—of these emotionally starved children home. But adults responding this way must remember: adoption is forever. If the baby has experienced severe deprivation or intrauterine exposure to toxins, alcohol, or drugs, the residual effects could also be forever. Adoptive parents need to be ready to love the baby they get, even if that baby is not the one they dreamed of.

In a province of South Korea, Taegu, a Presbyterian university had been built with funds from Texas. The president of Taegu University, Byongh Park had been to Boston to learn to use the NBAS with Kevin Nugent. Because of his experiences in Boston, they had erected a marble monument with my name on it. They got me to plant a cypress tree there. Among the other monuments were to President Carter, Eleanor Roosevelt, and Jacqueline and Jack Kennedy. I felt immortalized in Korea. A nice feeling, I suppose, but I wasn't dead yet.

Hong Kong completed our Asian tour. One of my ex-trainers, Dr. Lillian Koh, was in charge of NBAS training there. Lillian is a caring young woman who practices pediatrics and teaches in the medical school. Her husband, Hiao Cheng, was a successful urologist. Lillian has taught many people how to look at and to value babies. With her, we once again saw the quiet, gentle Asian newborns with their smoothly flowing motor activity. As we observed elsewhere, they rarely cry, and they don't build up to a lot of activity or loss of control. A fussy baby in this part of the world is unusual,

causing great concern to those around them. I noticed that everyone respected this high degree of sensitivity, speaking softly, and
rarely, if ever, got excited or demanding with them. They controlled
small children with quiet commands, never spanking or hitting. As
a result, these children seemed to learn by modeling—visual and
auditory, not by motor testing and exploration, like our children do
in the United States.

Children in War

A very different experience of advocacy abroad came in 1992.
James Grant, the dedicated CEO of UNICEF, called to ask me
whether I would be willing to go to Zagreb in Croatia with a
UNICEF group to see what we could do for the children who were
refugees from the fighting in Bosnia next door.

The war in Yugoslavia between Serbs and Bosnian Muslims
was raging. Sarajevo had turned from a bustling, Paris-like city into a
ravaged bomb site. The Serbs were in ascendance, the Muslims fleeing their homes. In the United States, we heard of the nightmares
that the victims of genocide were enduring, but it was far away. We
read about it, but our isolation afforded a kind of detachment.

Having never been offered such an opportunity, I agreed. But
my children heard about it. "Dad, are you crazy? You will be going
into the midst of a war! You are seventy-four. You'll be shot at, a
target for kidnapping. You just can't go." I was torn about whether
to listen to them, but moved by their concern. I called UNICEF to
tell them of my ambivalence. Jim Grant, by now, had assembled a
group of four of us "experts" and was unwilling to let me off the
hook. Secretly I was glad and looked forward to the adventure. My
children made me promise not to go to Sarajevo.

Zagreb, at that point, housed refugees from both sides and had not been bombed in the war. But it was surrounded by refugee camps and destitute, homeless survivors of the vicious attacks. As in the mass killings of Hitler's Germany or Pol Pot's Cambodia, the Balkans now bore witness to the racial genocide that seems to surface in cycles throughout history.

We began to hear about the mass rapes of the women and the torture and killing of men, young and old. The tales were hard to listen to, even harder to believe. Once Jim Grant had assembled us in our hotel in Zagreb, he began to plan a drive to Sarajevo to "see what really was happening and to try to contact the Serbian leaders to plead for their mercy for the children of Yugoslavia." The other three were ready to accompany Jim in a drive through the ravaged countryside to Sarajevo, several hundred miles from Zagreb. I had to insist on staying in Zagreb because I'd promised my children I wouldn't go. Jim Grant pleaded with me to come. I finally won out, full of guilt. When they returned safely a week later, it turned out that they had driven there in a little unprotected Volkswagen. It was now full of holes from being shot at. Mercifully, the group was unharmed, but they were completely discouraged and unsuccessful. Milošević was a fiend, and his pleasure in the genocide was evident to all of the international experts.

Meanwhile, I had turned my time into a productive set of visits to the refugee camps. With an interpreter, I was able to talk to the remnants of families left by this mass destruction. There were almost no men in the camps. One toothless old man pointed to himself and his ancient friend to say through a translator, "We are the only ones left." Many of the little girls had been raped repeatedly. They were terrified of me as a male and as a stranger. Few women had survived the mass rapes and the murders that followed. These Muslim women had been used to being veiled, protected in their households. This inflamed the invading Serbian armies. Little girls and early adolescent girls drew me vivid pictures of their assaults. Their faces were blank as if in shock. Their bodies stiff, they limped and wandered around as if in a daze.

One five-year-old boy was living in one of the shelter rooms with his grandmother. They were the only survivors of a large clan from a small town north of Zagreb. The five-year-old kept swatting flies away from his face. I commented to his grandmother that I didn't see any flies. She said, "Oh, no, they are just in his mind." She told me this story.

His young father was hiding in the cellar of their house when the Serbs invaded their village. A neighbor exposed the fact that there was a young male in hiding. The Serbs pulled him out, killed him in front of the family house, and hung him up by his hands to rot. The survivors were not allowed to bury their dead. The boy's young mother was too pregnant to rape so they cut her open to let her fetus fall out. Then they hung her up by her arms beside her husband. Both of these young people swung in front of the house, according to the grandmother. All the rest of the family was murdered. Meanwhile, this five-year-old had watched his dead parents through the screened front door. As they swung, flies gathered on the young woman's exposed fetus. The little boy sobbed out, "Keep away you flies. That's my baby, my baby." Ever since then he'd been batting flies away. The grandmother ended her tale by asking me, "Do you think he'll ever recover?" I couldn't reassure her. How could anyone ever recover from such horrors? Every child in this camp had a grim tale. This child was lucky to have one family member, his grandmother, left to care for him. Many didn't.

Each day held such nightmares. One day a young Italian social worker and psychologist, who was volunteering to try to help these people, recognized me and almost fell into my arms. "Dr. Brazelton, I've studied your work and have known about you for all of my professional life." She went on to say, "I'm burned out here. I try to get the children to go to school in Zagreb. They won't go. I get the surviving adults a job. They won't leave the camp to take the job. These people are so hopeless that I can't revive their spirits to get them to want to live again. It is burning me out. What do you do when you are burned out?"

I had never been confronted with such a question before. I tried to explain to her that the children couldn't dare to leave the adults with whom they had survived for fear that they'd never see them again. The adults couldn't take a job because it might symbolize the fact that they'd accepted their fate in fleeing from their homes. They all still had the fantasy that they'd be able to go home, sooner or later. She understood this. "But, what do you do for burnout?"

I blurted out, "I go see a newborn baby!" Her face brightened. She said, "I know of one who was just born. Can we go see him together?" Of course I agreed, and we proceeded across the camp to one of the huts where a young mother and her own mother were tending a newborn—a boy!

We asked permission to play with this miraculous young survivor in front of them. They were mesmerized when the baby turned to my voice, then chose his mother's voice over mine. His mother began to weep with joy. Without words, a new baby, once again, gave us all renewed courage and a feeling that the world might go on, in spite of the inhumanity of man to man.

Acknowledgments

Most of the people I want to thank are in the chapters of this memoir. All my colleagues at the Child Development Center and the Touchpoints Center have been supportive in the endeavors I have tried to record here.

Among those I would particularly like to acknowledge are my best friend and colleague Joshua Sparrow, who has been my mainstay for twenty-two years now and who will succeed me at the Touchpoints Center, and Kevin Nugent who has been so important in helping get the Neonatal Behavioral Assessment Scale in front of the public. I owe special thanks to Suzanne Otcasek, without whom I could not possibly manage. She helps me with all aspects of the work at the Touchpoints Center. Liz Wilson brought a lot of thought and care to typing the various versions of the manuscript. I am also indebted to my colleague Kyle Pruett and to Michelle Seaton, who read and commented on early drafts of the manuscript. My daughter Christina helped with each stage of the writing and, as always, with so much else.

Index

About the Author

T. Berry Brazelton, MD, founder of the Child Development Unit at Boston Children's Hospital, is Clinical Professor of Pediatrics Emeritus at Harvard Medical School and Professor of Pediatrics and Human Development at Brown University. He is also past president of the Society for Research in Child Development and of Zero to Three: The National Center for Infants, Toddlers, and Families. A practicing pediatrician for more than forty-five years, he introduced the concept of anticipatory guidance for parents into pediatric training. The author of more than two hundred scholarly papers, Dr. Brazelton has written thirty books for both professional and lay audiences, including *Touchpoints* (translated into eighteen languages), *To Listen to a Child*, and the now-classic trilogy *Infants and Mothers*, *Toddlers and Parents*, and *On Becoming a Family*. His television show, *What Every Baby Knows*, ran for twelve years and won an Emmy and three Ace Awards.

To continue his important research and implement its findings, Dr. Brazelton founded two programs at Boston Children's Hospital: the Brazelton Institute (furthering work with the Neonatal Behavioral Assessment Scale) and the Brazelton Touchpoints Center (training health and child care professionals across the country in the Touchpoints preventive outreach approach).

Among his very numerous awards, he is the recipient of the C. Anderson Aldrich Award for Distinguished Contributions to the Field of Child Development, given by the American Academy of Pediatrics, and the Woodrow Wilson Award for Outstanding Public Service from Princeton University. In 1988, Dr. Brazelton was appointed by the U.S. Congress to serve on the National Commission for Children, and in 2012 he was honored by the White House as a Head Start Champion of Change. Most recently, he received the prestigious 2012 Presidential Citizens Medal, awarded to those "who have performed exemplary deeds of service for their country or their fellow citizens."